Laboratory M

Editor

M. JANE MCDANIEL

PHYSICIAN ASSISTANT CLINICS

www.physicianassistant.theclinics.com

Consulting Editor
JAMES A. VAN RHEE

July 2019 • Volume 4 • Number 3

ELSEVIER

1600 John F. Kennedy Boulevard • Suite 1800 • Philadelphia, Pennsylvania, 19103-2899

http://www.theclinics.com

PHYSICIAN ASSISTANT CLINICS Volume 4, Number 3
July 2019 ISSN 2405-7991, ISBN-13: 978-0-323-67886-5

Editor: Jessica McCool
Developmental Editor: Casey Potter

Physician Assistant Clinics (ISSN: 2405–7991) is published quarterly by Elsevier Inc., 360 Park Avenue South, New York, NY 10010-1710. Months of issue are January, April, July, and October. Periodicals postage paid at New York, NY and additional mailing offices. Subscription prices are $150.00 per year (US individuals), $205.00 (US institutions), $100.00 (US students), $150.00 (Canadian individuals), $257.00 (Canadian institutions), $100.00 (Canadian students), $150.00 (international individuals), $257.00 (international institutions), and $100.00 (international students). Foreign air speed delivery is included in all *Clinics* subscription prices. All prices are subject to change without notice. POSTMASTER: Send address changes to *Physician Assistant Clinics*, Elsevier Periodicals Customer Service, 11830 Westline Industrial Drive, St. Louis, MO 63146. Customer Service Health Sciences Division, Subscription Customer Service, 3251 Riverport Lane, Maryland Heights, MO 63043. **Customer Service: 1-800-654-2452 (U.S. and Canada); 314-447-8871 (outside U.S. and Canada). Fax: 314-447-8029. E-mail: journalscustomerservice-usa@elsevier.com (for print support); journalsonlinesupport-usa@elsevier.com (for online support).**

Reprints. For copies of 100 or more, of articles in this publication, please contact the Commercial Reprints Department, Elsevier Inc., 360 Park Avenue South, New York, NY 10010-1710. Tel. 212-633-3874; Fax: 212-633-3820; E-mail: reprints@elsevier.com.

Physician Assistant Clinics is covered in *EMBASE/Excerpta Medica and ESCI.*

PROGRAM OBJECTIVE

The goal of the Physician Assistant Clinics is to keep practicing physician assistants up to date with current clinical practice by providing timely articles reviewing the state of the art in patient care.

TARGET AUDIENCE

Physician Assistants and other healthcare professionals.

LEARNING OBJECTIVES

Upon completion of this activity, participants will be able to:
1. Review anemia diagnostics and diagnostics for white blood cell abnormalities.
2. Discuss testing for renal, liver, and thyroid function.
3. Recognize new methods in dementia testing.

ACCREDITATION

The Elsevier Office of Continuing Medical Education (EOCME) is accredited by the Accreditation Council for Continuing Medical Education (ACCME) to provide continuing medical education for physicians.

The EOCME designates this enduring material for a maximum of 15 *AMA PRA Category 1 Credit*(s)™. Physicians should claim only the credit commensurate with the extent of their participation in the activity.

All other health care professionals requesting continuing education credit for this enduring material will be issued a certificate of participation.

DISCLOSURE OF CONFLICTS OF INTEREST

The EOCME assesses conflict of interest with its instructors, faculty, planners, and other individuals who are in a position to control the content of CME activities. All relevant conflicts of interest that are identified are thoroughly vetted by EOCME for fair balance, scientific objectivity, and patient care recommendations. EOCME is committed to providing its learners with CME activities that promote improvements or quality in healthcare and not a specific proprietary business or a commercial interest.

The planning committee, staff, authors and editors listed below have identified no financial relationships or relationships to products or devices they or their spouse/life partner have with commercial interest related to the content of this CME activity:
Carey L. Barry, MHS, PA-C, MT(ASCP); Kathleen Barta, PA-C, MPAS; Debra A. Herrmann, DHSc, MPH, PA-C; Casey Jackson; Alison Kemp; Mary Jean Leonardi, MAT, MMS, PA-C; Patricia G. Martin, BS-MT (ASCP), MBA, PA-C; Jessica McCool; M. Jane McDaniel, MS, MLS(ASCP)SC; Jason Parente, MS, PA-C; Dipu Patel, MPAS, PA-C; Molly Paulson, DHSc, MPAS, PA-C, MT (ASCP), DFAAPA; Robert Paxton, PA-C, MPAS; Arunkumar Rangarajan; Benjamin J Smith, MPAS, PA-C, DFAAPA; Annamarie Faust Streilein, MT(ASCP), MHS, PA-C; James A. Van Rhee, MS, PA-C; Joshua L. Waynick, MMS, PA-C.

The planning committee, staff, authors and editors listed below have identified financial relationships or relationships to products or devices they or their spouse/life partner have with commercial interest related to the content of this CME activity:
Erik Munson, Ph.D., D(ABMM): receives research support from Hologic Inc.

UNAPPROVED/OFF-LABEL USE DISCLOSURE

The EOCME requires CME faculty to disclose to the participants:
1. When products or procedures being discussed are off-label, unlabelled, experimental, and/or investigational (not US Food and Drug Administration [FDA] approved); and
2. Any limitations on the information presented, such as data that are preliminary or that represent ongoing research, interim analyses, and/or unsupported opinions. Faculty may discuss information about pharmaceutical agents that is outside of FDA-approved labelling. This information is intended solely for CME and is not intended to promote off-label use of these medications. If you have any questions, contact the medical affairs department of the manufacturer for the most recent prescribing information.

TO ENROLL

The CME program is available to all Physician Assistant Clinics subscribers at no additional fee. To subscribe to the Physician Assistant Clinics, call customer service at 1-800-654-2452 or sign up online at www.physicianassistant.theclinics.com.

METHOD OF PARTICIPATION

In order to claim credit, participants must complete the following:

1. Complete enrolment as indicated above.
2. Read the activity.
3. Complete the CME Test and Evaluation. Participants must achieve a score of 70% on the test. All CME Tests and Evaluations must be completed online.

CME INQUIRIES/SPECIAL NEEDS

For all CME inquiries or special needs, please contact elsevierCME@elsevier.com.

Contributors

CONSULTING EDITOR

JAMES A. VAN RHEE, MS, PA-C
Associate Professor, Program Director, Yale School of Medicine, Yale Physician Assistant Online Program, New Haven, Connecticut

EDITOR

M. JANE McDANIEL, MS, MLS(ASCP)SC
Lecturer, Yale School of Medicine, Yale Physician Assistant Online Program, New Haven, Connecticut

AUTHORS

CAREY L. BARRY, MHS, PA-C, MT(ASCP)
Assistant Clinical Professor, Physician Assistant Program, Northeastern University, Boston, Massachusetts

KATHLEEN BARTA, PA-C, MPAS
Physician Assistant, Infectious Disease Specialists of Southeastern Wisconsin, Brookfield, Wisconsin

DEBRA A. HERRMANN, DHSc, MPH, PA-C
Assistant Professor, Department of Physician Assistant Studies, The George Washington University, Washington, DC

MARY JEAN LEONARDI, MAT, MMS, PA-C
Instructor, Physician Assistant Program, Department of PA Studies, Wake Forest School of Medicine, Winston-Salem, North Carolina

PATRICIA G. MARTIN, BS-MT (ASCP), MBA, PA-C
Assistant Professor, Retired, Physician Assistant Program, Marietta College, Marietta, Ohio

M. JANE McDANIEL, MS, MLS(ASCP)SC
Lecturer, Yale School of Medicine, Yale Physician Assistant Online Program, New Haven, Connecticut

ERIK MUNSON, PhD, D(ABMM)
Assistant Professor, Department of Clinical Laboratory Science, College of Health Sciences, Marquette University, Milwaukee, Wisconsin

JASON PARENTE, MS, PA-C
Assistant Clinical Professor, Physician Assistant Program, Northeastern University, Boston, Massachusetts

DIPU PATEL, MPAS, PA-C
Associate Program Director, Director of Simulation Education, Assistant Clinical Professor, Northeastern University PA Program, Boston, Massachusetts

MOLLY PAULSON, DHSc, MPAS, PA-C, MT (ASCP), DFAAPA
Assistant Professor of Physician Assistant Studies, College of Health Professions, Grand Valley State University, Grand Rapids, Michigan

ROBERT PAXTON, PA-C, MPAS
Associate Director, Director of Didactic Education, Department of Physician Assistant Studies, College of Health Sciences, Marquette University, Milwaukee, Wisconsin

BENJAMIN J SMITH, MPAS, PA-C, DFAAPA
Director of Didactic Education, Assistant Professor, Florida State University College of Medicine School of Physician Assistant Practice, Tallahassee, Florida

ANNAMARIE FAUST STREILEIN, MT(ASCP), MHS, PA-C
Director of Preclinical Education, Duke Physician Assistant Program, Assistant Professor, Department of Family Medicine and Community Health, Duke University Medical Center, Durham, North Carolina; Physician Assistant, Alamance County Health Department, Burlington, North Carolina

JAMES A. VAN RHEE, MS, PA-C
Associate Professor, Program Director, Yale School of Medicine, Yale Physician Assistant Online Program, New Haven, Connecticut

JOSHUA L. WAYNICK, MMS, PA-C
Instructor, Department of PA Studies, Wake Forest School of Medicine, Winston-Salem, North Carolina

Contents

Rheumatology laboratory testing can induce anxiety for both patients and medical providers. Health care professionals, including physician assistants, are often perplexed by the laboratory testing needed to diagnose and monitor rheumatic disease. The question of which laboratory test to order, when to order which test, and what to do with the results is common. Screening diagnostic laboratory tests, including rheumatoid factors and antinuclear antibodies are important serologic tests, but other rheumatic disease-associated laboratory tests are available. A strategic approach is described for ordering rheumatology laboratory tests, enabling clinicians to have confidence when caring for persons with rheumatic conditions.

In this article, we review the use of nucleic acid amplification testing as it specifically applies to diagnosing the following sexually transmitted infections (STIs): *Neisseria gonorrhoeae, Chlamydia trachomatis, Mycoplasma genitalium*, and *Trichomonas vaginalis*. The use of molecular testing for nonulcerative STI has led to decreased time to diagnosis, improved sensitivity and specificity of previous testing methods, and more rapid treatment by clinicians. Clinicians need to be aware of the most recent updates in testing methods as well as the limits of the laboratory used for testing.

This article reviews cardiac troponin with an emphasis on anatomy, physiology, process of obtaining the level, differential diagnosis, and interpretation within the clinical context as well as novel markers for cardiac myocyte damage. Natriuretic peptides are discussed with a focus on anatomy, physiology, process of obtaining the level, differential diagnosis, clinical scenarios, and patient factors that make interpretation difficult.

Thyroid disease is frequently encountered by clinicians. Symptoms are multifactorial, overlap with, and confound, other medical conditions. This makes thyroid testing an essential component in the investigation of many disease processes. Clinicians must have a clear understanding of thyroid physiology, identify when testing is indicated, order appropriate tests, and know how to interpret the test results based on the patient's presenting symptoms and comorbidities.

Evaluation of hepatic function testing is crucial to the detection and diagnosis of hepatobiliary disease because specific patterns of elevations in the basic hepatic function tests can aid in the differentiation of prehepatic, hepatic, and posthepatic organ involvement. A detailed patient history should be obtained and basic hepatic function laboratory tests, such as fractionated bilirubin, aspartate aminotransferase, alanine aminotransferase, alkaline phosphatase, and γ-glutamyl transferase, should direct clinicians to additional testing that can aid in a final diagnosis. This article outlines an approach to patients with elevated hepatic function tests and reviews the common etiologies and diagnostic testing protocols.

The correct interpretation of arterial blood gas (ABG) results requires an understanding of acid-base balance. The body's regulation of pH is influenced by the respiratory and metabolic systems; bicarbonate (HCO_3) represents the metabolic influence, and partial pressure of carbon dioxide ($Paco_2$) represents the respiratory influence. The pH is dependent on the $Paco_2/HCO_3$ ratio. A change in $Paco_2$ is compensated by a shift in HCO_3 and vice versa. This review outlines a 6-step plan for ABG interpretation informed by an evaluation of multiple strategies. Three case studies illustrate use of the 6-step ABG interpretation process.

This article discusses laboratory studies, which assist the clinician in assessing renal health. Current guidelines and the newest recommendations on when and who to test are examined. Focus is placed on the use of urinalysis and estimated glomerular filtration rate to screen and stage chronic kidney disease, the use of creatinine and noncreatinine biomarkers to detect acute kidney injury, the advantages of urine protein and urine electrolyte analysis in establishing underlying pathologic condition, and the use of imaging and biopsy to confirm diagnosis and underlying pathologic condition.

 Video content accompanies this article at http://www. physicianassistant.theclinics.com.

This article provides an overview of provider-performed microscopy (PPM) procedures approved by the Clinical Laboratory Improvement

Amendment. Benefits of PPM procedures are discussed, as are regulations and requirements for their performance by clinicians. A summary of the 9 PPM procedures is provided and includes microscopic findings, test principles, and their diagnostic utility.

Immunohematology is the foundation of transfusion medicine. Immunohematology and the fundamentals of blood banking are examined, including ABO, Rh, and minor blood typing, antibody screening, crossmatching, Coombs testing, and blood product compatibility. Current recommendations for packed red blood cell, platelet, and fresh frozen plasma transfusion are reviewed.

Hemostasis requires a complex system of procoagulation and anticoagulation processes that allow for rapid clot formation in an area of blood vessel damage but prevent inappropriate or excessive clot formation. Imbalances or disruptions in this system that favor anticoagulation can lead to excessive bleeding. Imbalances that favor procoagulation can lead to clot development that occludes arteries or veins. Evaluation of a person with impaired hemostasis requires a thorough history and physical examination. These findings guide selection of appropriate laboratory diagnostics. This article reviews the basic processes of hemostasis and outlines available diagnostics to identify underlying causes of bleeding and clotting disorders.

This article defines common terminology in the evaluation of the complete blood count, specifically as it relates to leukocytosis and leukopenia. Common etiologies are explored and diagnostic approaches are provided.

Presentation of patients to the primary care setting with anemia is fairly common. Therefore, understanding the treatment and management of anemia is imperative for any physician assistant practice. Interpreting the complete blood cell count in the context of a clinical presentation aids in improving patient outcomes and treatment of common complaints. The presentation of anemia can be vague and, therefore, the index of suspicion must be high. Furthermore, deeper understanding of the red blood cell cycle and the various organs involved helps in appropriate and cost-effective work-up of anemia.

Hemolytic anemias may be acute or chronic and life-threatening. They should be considered in all patients with an unexplained normocytic or macrocytic anemia. A detailed history should be obtained and basic laboratory tests, such as lactate dehydrogenase, indirect bilirubin, haptoglobin, and reticulocyte count, and review of the peripheral blood smear should direct clinicians to more specific tests that can aid in the diagnosis. This article provides an approach to patients with hemolytic anemia and reviews the common etiologies.

PHYSICIAN ASSISTANT CLINICS

SERIES OF RELATED INTEREST

Clinics in Laboratory Medicine
https://www.labmed.theclinics.com/

THE CLINICS ARE AVAILABLE ONLINE!
Access your subscription at:
www.theclinics.com

Foreword
Laboratory Medicine

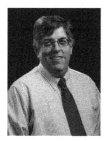

James A. Van Rhee, MS, PA-C
Consulting Editor

Thirty-seven years ago, I finished my training as a medical technologist and started a career working in the lab. The career was fairly short, as a few years later I started PA school. What I did take with me from my medical technology days was a respect for the lab and an understanding of how the lab works, how to interpret labs, and what to order when. Since not everyone can get medical technology training prior to starting PA school, I hope this issue of *Physician Assistant Clinics* can possibly substitute for that lack of training. At least a little bit, I hope.

The guest editor, M. Jane McDaniel, has put together an excellent group of clinicians, some with training in medical technology prior to becoming physician assistants, to provide you with the latest in laboratory medicine.

The complete blood count is one of the most commonly ordered tests in clinical practice. White blood cell abnormalities are reviewed by Parente; anemia diagnostics is covered by Patel, and yours truly covers the evaluation of hemolytic anemias. To finish off hematology, Barry provides information related to transfusion medicine, and Leonardi reviews the evaluation of the hemostatic disorders.

Clinical chemistry is covered by McDaniel, who provides the ABCs of liver function tests; Martin reviews renal function testing, and Herrmann demystifies arterial blood gases. Cardiac markers are discussed by Waynick; Paulson reviews thyroid testing, and Smith describes how rheumatology tests can be used in diagnosing rheumatic disease.

There have been advances in microbiology testing, and Paxton provides an update in the new procedures used in diagnosing sexually transmitted disease. If you do any microscopy in your office, Streilein provides an excellent review with some great photos reviewing the more common office-performed microscopy procedures.

Physician Assist Clin 4 (2019) xiii–xiv
https://doi.org/10.1016/j.cpha.2019.03.002
2405-7991/19/© 2019 Published by Elsevier Inc.

physicianassistant.theclinics.com

I hope you enjoy this issue. This issue brought me back to those days I worked in the laboratory, but I can tell you, things have really changed. Our next issue will provide you with a review of the latest in Disaster Medicine.

James A. Van Rhee, MS, PA-C
Yale School of Medicine
Yale Physician Assistant Online Program
100 Church Street South, Suite A230
New Haven, CT 06519, USA

E-mail address:
james.vanrhee@yale.edu

Website:
http://www.paonline.yale.edu

Preface

Blazing New Trails in Laboratory Medicine

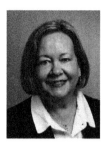

M. Jane McDaniel, MS, MLS(ASCP)SC
Editor

Laboratory Medicine is one of the most rapidly changing fields in medicine. In every specialty, the protocol for ordering diagnostic testing is constantly changing due to the addition of new and improved diagnostic tests. Some of these diagnostic tests are better simply because they have greater sensitivity and/or specificity. Other diagnostic tests are designed to measure a newly identified marker or substance that has not been previously tested. And still other diagnostic tests are developed due to new research or clinical guidelines that alter previously identified norms. Whatever the reason for the development of these new and improved diagnostic tests, keeping abreast of the latest technology can be challenging.

One of the areas of medicine that many clinicians find particularly challenging is the ordering and interpretation of rheumatology laboratory tests. Keeping up with the most up-to-date diagnostic tests in this category can be extremely perplexing, which is why we have attempted to provide an update of the newest tests available as well as a strategic approach to ordering and interpreting these tests, thus improving clinician confidence in caring for these patients.

Another area that is rapidly changing and evolving in the field of laboratory medicine is the testing involved in diagnosing sexually transmitted infections. The move to increased molecular testing in this area of laboratory medicine has led to improved turn-around time for diagnosis, resulting in more rapid treatment. As a result, clinicians can provide better patient care in a more condensed timeframe.

There are many other areas of diagnostic testing that are rapidly evolving, including cardiac marker testing, thyroid testing, coagulation testing, and transfusion medicine testing. Each of these areas is presented by it respective authors with an emphasis on the latest diagnostic tests available as well as the guidelines for interpreting these diagnostic tests. Our hope is that clinicians will find these up-to-date articles extremely helpful as they work to update their patient care regimens.

Physician Assist Clin 4 (2019) xv–xvi
https://doi.org/10.1016/j.cpha.2019.03.001
2405-7991/19/© 2019 Published by Elsevier Inc.

physicianassistant.theclinics.com

In addition to the newer, more advanced laboratory medicine technologies that are available, clinicians also have a need to better understand some of the more traditional diagnostic test methods and results that are presented in our articles on provider-performed microscopy testing, renal function testing, arterial blood gas testing and interpretation, and hepatic function testing. These articles reinforce clinician understanding of some of the basic elements of laboratory testing while stimulating clinical reasoning skills in interpreting results.

Hematology testing for blood cell disorders and interpretation of complete blood count results is the final area of laboratory medicine that we will cover and one that can be challenging. From white blood cell abnormalities to the various anemias and red blood cell abnormalities, we strive to help you better understand these disease processes as well as the laboratory testing that defines them in order to enhance quality patient care.

As the guest editor of this Laboratory Medicine issue of *Physician Assistant Clinics*, I am thrilled to introduce you to the extremely talented individuals who authored each of these articles and provided you with some insight into their laboratory medicine areas of expertise. Our goal is to improve your understanding of all of these state-of-the-art test methodologies to help you better care for your patients.

M. Jane McDaniel, MS, MLS(ASCP)SC
Yale School of Medicine
Physician Assistant Online Program
100 Church Street South, Suite A230
New Haven, CT 06519, USA

E-mail address:
jane.mcdaniel@yale.edu

Website:
http://www.paonline.yale.edu

Rheumatology Laboratory Tests

A Piece of the Rheumatic Disease Diagnostic Puzzle

Benjamin J Smith, MPAS, PA-C, DFAAPA

KEYWORDS

- Rheumatology • Laboratory • Rheumatoid factor • Anticyclic citrillunated antibody
- Antinuclear antibody • HLA-B27

KEY POINTS

- The appropriate use of laboratory diagnostics is vital when caring for those with rheumatic disease.
- Antinuclear antibodies, rheumatoid factors, and cyclic citrullinated peptides are helpful diagnostic laboratory, but are not used to measure disease activity.
- The immunofluorescence antinuclear antibody test is the gold standard for antinuclear antibody testing.
- When ordering a rheumatoid factor test, consider also ordering a cyclic citrullinated peptide test.

Rheumatic disease is prevalent. Many rheumatic conditions are systemic and inflammatory in nature. Because these disorders have the potential to affect multiple body organs and can present suddenly or insidiously, diagnosing these conditions can be challenging. This diagnostic uncertainty can lead to increased patient anxiety and the need for health care providers to be constantly considering the differential diagnosis. Although laboratory studies do not provide a definitive diagnosis in and of themselves, appropriately selected laboratory tests can aid in making a rheumatic disease diagnosis. Laboratory testing is one piece of the diagnostic puzzle.

This article discusses the diagnostic serologies and monitoring laboratory tests that assist health care providers in caring for persons with rheumatic disease. The structure of this article is to discuss laboratory tests specific to common rheumatic conditions treated by physician assistants as noted in a recent survey.[1] These conditions

Disclosure Statement: None.
Florida State University College of Medicine School of Physician Assistant Practice, 1115 West Call Street, Tallahassee, FL 32306-4300, USA
E-mail address: benjamin.smith@med.fsu.edu

Physician Assist Clin 4 (2019) 487–500
https://doi.org/10.1016/j.cpha.2019.02.002
2405-7991/19/© 2019 Elsevier Inc. All rights reserved.

include the following: rheumatoid arthritis (RA), systemic lupus erythematosus (SLE), Sjogren syndrome, progressive systemic sclerosis, seronegative spondyloarthropathies, gout, vasculitis, polymyalgia rheumatica (PMR)/giant cell arteritis (GCA), inflammatory myopathies, fibromyalgia, and osteoarthritis (OA).

REVIEW OF BIOSTATISTICAL TERMS

In a discussion of how to interpret laboratory results, a brief review of biostatistical terms is warranted. **Table 1** lists important terms and definitions to consider when evaluating the performance of a diagnostic test. **Table 2** provides a guide to calculating usefulness of diagnostic tests.

LABORATORY RESULTS AS PART OF THE DIAGNOSTIC PUZZLE

Like those who work in other medical specialties, those who treat persons with rheumatic disease must use each piece of the puzzle to most effectively care for persons whom they serve. The puzzle comes together when health care providers hear what patients say and recognize how they communicate their experiences, observe features of a person's presentation, and use available ancillary resources such as laboratory and radiographic studies. In other words, the pieces of the puzzle include obtaining a through history including past medical history and review of systems, performing a skilled physical examination, and ordering and interpreting laboratory and radiographic studies.

Sensitivities and specificities for rheumatology serologies are not 100%. This means that some patients with a given disease will have negative serologies and persons without a given condition will have positive serologies. A review of the literature shows that 20% to 30% of persons with RA are seronegative for rheumatoid factor (RF) and/or anti–cyclic citrullinated peptide (CCP).[2,3] Seronegative SLE has also been described in the medical literature representing 1% to 5% of persons with SLE having a negative antinuclear antibody (ANA).[4–9] Seroconversion may occur later in the disease course.

Conversely, patients may present with positive serologies not manifesting signs or symptoms of clinical disease. Studies have demonstrated the formation of antibodies years before the onset of clinical disease.[10–12] Currently, there are no validated measures or treatments that prevent the onset of RA and SLE. A reasonable approach that rheumatology health providers use is to follow patients with positive serologies

Table 1
Biostatistical terms and definitions

Sensitivity	The true positive rate, number of patients with a positive test who have the disease divided by all of the patients who have the disease.
Specificity	The true negative rate, number of patients with a negative test who do not have the disease divided by all of the patients who do not have the disease.
Positive predictive value	Likelihood that a patient with a positive result has the disease, dependent on disease prevalence in a population.
Negative predictive value	Likelihood that a patient with a negative result does not have the disease, dependent on disease prevalence in a population.
Likelihood ratios	Odds of having a disease relative to prior probability of the disease.

Table 2 Determining sensitivity, specificity, predictive values and likelihood ratios		
	Disease Present	Disease Absent
Test result (+)	A	B
Test result (−)	C	D
Sensitivity = A/(A + C)		
Specificity = D/(B + D)		
Positive predictive value = A/(A + B)		
Negative predictive value = D/(C + D)		
Positive likelihood ratio = sensitivity/(1 − specificity)		
Negative likelihood ratio = (1 − sensitivity)/specificity		

without clinical disease serially with follow-up visits every 6 to 12 months or with any change in signs or symptoms.

RHEUMATOID ARTHRITIS

RA is a chronic, systemic, inflammatory arthritis that primarily affects peripheral synovial joints. Extraarticular manifestations may occur with RA, including potential affects to bone, skin, eyes, lung, heart, blood vessels, and blood. The 2 most common diagnostic laboratory tests for RA are RF and anti–citrullinated peptide antibodies (ACPA).

Rheumatoid Factor

Waaler and Rose first described RF in the 1940s.[13] RF is an autoantibody directed against the Fc portion of immunoglobulin G. RF may be of various isotypes (IgG, IgA, IgM, IgE), but IgM is the most commonly tested. There are various techniques used in the laboratory to test for RF: nephelometry, enzyme-linked immunosorbent assay, and latex agglutination techniques. The sensitivity and specificity of RF for RA are 50% to 80% and 80% to 90%, respectively.[13]

RF is a diagnostic laboratory test and should not be used to measure disease activity at a given point in time. For this reason, ordering serial RFs is not recommended. Persons with a higher titer RF have a greater potential for more severe disease, including articular and extraarticular manifestations. If a person has suspected seronegative RA, it is reasonable to order an RF periodically because patients with RA do seroconvert during the course of the disease.

RF positivity may occur in conditions other than RA. The mnemonic CHRONIC[14] assists health care providers in recognizing when a positive RF is associated when non-RA diagnosis.

CH: Chronic disease (especially hepatic and pulmonary diseases);
R: Rheumatoid arthritis;
O: Other rheumatic diseases (such as SLE, systemic sclerosis, mixed connective tissue disease, Sjogren syndrome, polymyositis, and sarcoidosis);
N: Neoplasms;
I: Infections (eg, AIDS, mononucleosis, parasitic infections, chronic viral infections including hepatitis B, hepatitis C, chronic bacterial infections, syphilis, and mycobacterial infections; and
C: Cryoglobulinemia (especially with hepatitis C).

Anti–Citrullinated Peptide Antibodies

ACPA is the most recent clinically available diagnostic laboratory associated with RA. The most common ACPA is anti-CCP antibodies. Anti-CCP has a similar sensitivity for RA as does the RF, but the specificity is 96%,[15] which serves as a great tool when considering the diagnosis in a person with inflammatory joint symptoms.

Like RF, anti-CCP can be associated with other rheumatic and nonrheumatic conditions. These conditions include SLE, primary Sjogren syndrome, psoriatic arthritis, and active tuberculosis. A positive anti-CCP is less commonly seen in persons with hepatitis C. Knowing that RF can be positive with hepatitis C, a result of a negative anti-CCP may lead a clinician to consider investigating for hepatitis C in the appropriate clinical scenario. As with RF, a positive anti-CCP is associated with potentially increased risk of destructive or erosive RA. A positive RF and anti-CCP may lead a provider to be more aggressive with pharmacologic treatment to prevent degenerative and debilitating joint changes.

The medical literature does suggest that RF and anti-CCP can be positive in persons before the onset of clinical disease. Nielen and colleagues[12] describe finding these autoantibodies a median of 4.5 years before symptom onset. Following a patient with positive RF and anti-CCP without clinical manifestations, after other diagnoses have been ruled out, is reasonable. Asking patients to contact their health care provider with any change of symptoms suggestive of inflammatory arthritis is encouraged.

The Vectra-DA test and the IdentRA test can be used for RA disease monitoring and for prognostic purposes. Although these tests are available, they have a low use by health care providers when compared with RF and anti-CCP.

SYSTEMIC LUPUS ERYTHEMATOSUS

SLE is an inflammatory, multisystem, autoimmune disease of unknown etiology with protean clinical and laboratory manifestations and a variable course and prognosis. Persons diagnosed with SLE may have a very mild presentation or may present with aggressive and life-threatening disease. Laboratory studies are tremendously helpful in both diagnosing and monitoring disease activity.

The ANA is the most common laboratory test associated with SLE, but other serologies aid in treating persons with SLE, which are further discussed elsewhere in this article.

Antinuclear Antibody

Hargraves[16] first described lupus erythematosus cells in sera of patients with SLE in 1948. There are numerous methods for detecting ANA in the laboratory: immunofluorescent microscopy, immunodiffusion, hemagglutination, complement fixation, solid phase immunoassay (enzyme-linked immunosorbent assay or immunoblotting), and radioimmunoassays. The American College of Rheumatology (ACR) has published a position statement stating that the immunofluorescence ANA testing using human epithelial type 2 substrate is the gold standard when ordering an ANA.[17] This technique, when it yields a positive result, yields a titer and pattern. Numerous studies support this position by the ACR.[18–21] Like RF in RA, a positive ANA can be associated with conditions other than SLE. **Box 1** lists other conditions associated with a positive ANA, both rheumatic and nonrheumatic diseases.

ANA titers provide a strength of positivity of the result. Lower titer ANA results are more commonly associated with false-positive results, whereas higher titer ANA results are more likely to be associated with clinical disease.[22,23] It is of upmost

---

Box 1
Diseases associated with a positive ANA

SLE

Progressive systemic sclerosis

RA

Sjogren syndrome

Mixed connective tissue disease

Drug-associated lupus

Raynaud phenomenon

Polymyositis/dermatomyositis

Juvenile chronic arthritis, with uveitis

Thyroid disease

Multiple sclerosis

Autoimmune hepatitis

Infectious disease

Idiopathic thrombocytopenic purpura

Fibromyalgia

Malignancies

Spondylarthropathies

Miscellaneous other conditions

Data from Solomon DH, Kavanaugh AJ, Schur, et al. Evidence-based guidelines for the use of immunologic tests: antinuclear antibody testing. Arthritis Rheum 2002;47(4):434–44.

---

importance that clinicians use the ANA result as one piece of the clinical puzzle. A positive ANA result is not in and of itself confirmatory of a diagnosis of SLE or any other autoimmune disorder.

Like RF, a positive ANA result may precede the onset of clinical disease.[10,11] Asking a patient with a moderately elevated ANA titer or greater to follow-up periodically, perhaps every 6 to 12 months, or with the onset of new symptoms suggestive of systemic autoimmunity is a reasonable approach. Patient education is key, because positive laboratory test results without clinical symptoms often lead to patient questions. Some patients with a positive ANA never develop clinical manifestations of SLE, other autoimmune disease, or other conditions.[22]

Health care providers will often ask the meaning of the ANA pattern that is provided as a result when the immunofluorescent laboratory technique is used for ANA determination. Various staining patterns are possible—namely, speckled, nucleolar, diffuse, and centromere. Generally, the ANA pattern is not helpful as a diagnostic aid, except the centromere patterned ANA. A centromere pattern can be associated with the CREST syndrome, or limited cutaneous systemic sclerosis. The acronym CREST represents the manifestations associated with this condition: Calcinosis, Raynaud phenomenon, Esophageal dysfunction, Sclerodactyly, and Telangiectasias. Some patients may have 2 ANA patterns, which also makes the result less likely to be a false positive. Because ANAs are not a measure of disease activity, serially ordering ANAs is not an effective use of health care resources.

Other Lupus Serologies

Although ANA is the most common laboratory test associated with SLE, other laboratory tests can be supportive of a lupus diagnosis or used for monitoring disease activity.

Lupus diagnostic serologies

Extractable nuclear antibodies When an extractable nuclear antibody test is ordered, the results often result in an anti-Smith (anti-Sm) and an anti-U1 ribonucleoprotein (anti-U1 RNP). Autoantigens to Ro (SS-A) and La (SS-B) are also extractable nuclear antibodies and are discussed elsewhere in the article in the Sjogren syndrome section.

The anti-Sm is very specific for the diagnosis of SLE. Anti-Sm sensitivity for SLE is 10% to 50% and specificity is 55% to 100%.[24–26] SLE patients with a positive anti-Sm may be younger at age of diagnosis and may be more prone to renal disease.

Of patients with SLE, 3% to 69% may be found with anti-U1 RNP positivity. Anti-U1 RNP is present in all patients with mixed connective tissue disease. Mixed connective tissue disease is a well-defined, overlap autoimmune condition that includes features of SLE, systemic sclerosis, and polymyositis, together with a high titer anti-U1 RNP. Other serologies, like ANA, may also be positive in patients with mixed connective tissue disease.

Lupus disease monitoring serologies

System review laboratory studies such as complete blood counts and comprehensive metabolic panels are helpful to screen for organ dysfunction. Renal function screening can also be accomplished with urinalysis, and, when indicated, other urine studies such as a 24-hour urine collection for protein or a protein/creatinine ratio to further quantitate kidney function or proteinuria.

Double-stranded DNA is of benefit because its presence has a high specificity for SLE activity, specifically lupus nephritis. As a disease monitoring laboratory test, double-stranded DNA is helpful when one suspects increased disease activity. An increasing double-stranded DNA level can be indicative of increased disease activity. Single-stranded DNA is generally not a useful laboratory test because it does not correlate with clinical activity.

Complements are a part of the innate immune system. Complements serve several functions in the immune system, including the promotion of inflammation. The commonly ordered complements in clinical rheumatology practice are CH50, C3, and C4. CH50, or the total hemolytic complement, is useful for detecting a deficiency in the classical pathway, whether from an inherited process or secondary to disease-related process. C3 and C4 are helpful when considering SLE activity, but may also be reduced in antiphospholipid syndrome, mixed cryoglobulinemia, Sjogren syndrome, subacute bacterial endocarditis, bacterial sepsis, hepatitis B, parasitemias, and post-streptococcal glomerulonephritis. A low CH50, C3, or C4 may indicate disease activity, whereas complement ranges that return to a normal range may be suggestive of response to treatment or decreased flare of disease.

Although non-ANA serologies are important diagnostic and monitoring factors, they should be ordered when clinically appropriate. The ACR's *Choosing Wisely* campaign included a recommendation that ANA subserologies should not be ordered without a positive ANA or without the clinical suspicion for a rheumatic disease.[27]

SJOGREN SYNDROME

Sjogren syndrome is a chronic, autoimmune, inflammatory condition for which patients often present with dryness of the eyes and mouth. The manifestations of Sjogren is often described as glandular or extraglandular in nature. Extraglandular features of Sjogren may affect multiple organ systems.

SS-A and SS-B are laboratory studies commonly associate with Sjogren syndrome. Of patients with Sjogren syndrome, 60% to 80% will have a positive test for one or both of these serologies. SS-A and SS-B are generally ordered together. Females who are in their childbearing years with a positive SS-A should discuss this finding with their obstetrician because a positive SS-A can be associated with congenital heart block or neonatal lupus. Referral to a high-risk obstetrician is often considered.

SYSTEMIC SCLEROSIS

Systemic sclerosis is a rheumatic disease that is often referred to by the term sclero-derma, which is one manifestation of the condition. As with other inflammatory rheu-matic diseases, systemic involvement can occur.

Antitopoisomerase I is laboratory test associated with systemic sclerosis. Those pa-tients with systemic sclerosis with a positive antitopoisomerase I are more likely to have severe interstitial lung disease. An ANA is found in 95% of patients with systemic sclerosis.[28] Even with positive laboratory studies, systemic sclerosis is often a diag-nosis based on the physical examination.

SERONEGATIVE SPONDYLOARTHROPATHIES

The family of arthritis disease entities called seronegative spondyloarthropathy in-cludes axial spondyloarthritis, psoriatic arthritis, enteropathic arthritis (or inflammatory bowel disease associated with arthritis), and reactive arthritis. Axial spondylarthritis is further described as ankylosing spondylitis classified as those with sacroiliitis on plain film and nonradiographic axial spondyloarthritis in those who do not demonstrate plain film changes consistent with sacroiliitis. Patients with seronegative spondyloarthropa-thies may have articular or periarticular symptoms, including synovitis, enthesitis, or dactylitis. Extraarticular manifestations of seronegative spondyloarthropathies may include uveitis, psoriasis, or inflammatory bowel disease. Cardiac, pulmonary, and renal signs may also be present, although are much less common. HLA-B27 is the gene most commonly associated with seronegative spondyloarthropathies and is readily available in clinical settings.

HLA-B27

When a health care provider has a high degree of suspicion for a seronegative spon-dyloarthropathy, diagnostic laboratory tests may not be required. In North America, HLA-B27 is found in 6% to 9% of healthy Caucasians and 3% of healthy African Amer-icans. Only 2% of HLA-B27–positive individuals develop ankylosing spondylitis in their lifetime, although this increases to 15% to 20% if a first-degree relative has ankylosing spondylitis. HLA-B27 is found in 85% to 95% of Caucasian persons with ankylosing spondylitis[29,30] and 75 to 85% of persons with nonradiographic spondyloarthritis.[31–33] Similar to other diagnostic rheumatic disease laboratory studies, HLA-B27 is neither 100% sensitive or specific for seronegative spondyloarthropathy. However, the detec-tion of HLA-B27 may support a clinician's suspicion in cases of undifferentiated in-flammatory polyarthritis or inflammatory back pain symptoms.

GOUT

Monosodium urate crystal deposition disease is commonly known as gout. Gout is the most common inflammatory arthritis in men over the age of 40 and does not commonly occur in premenopausal women. Owing to the increase in obesity, the metabolic syndrome, and the use of medications like aspirin and diuretics, the prevalence of gout has increased in recent decades. Although gout is commonly recognized as an inflammatory arthropathy, clinicians must also be aware of potential extraarticular or comorbid conditions associated with gout, namely, hypertension, dyslipidemia, atherosclerosis, and glucose intolerance. Serum uric acid is the most common laboratory associated with gout.

Serum Uric Acid

Although the definitive diagnosis of gout is made by noting monosodium urate crystals in synovial fluid, obtaining a serum uric acid can aid in supporting the diagnosis of gout and assist in monitoring the course of the disease. During a gout flare, the serum uric acid level may be high, low, or normal. The ideal time to order a serum uric acid to obtain the clearest picture of a patient's serum uric acid level is during an intercritical period of gout activity. Also, serum uric acid should also be obtained after the initiation of urate lowering medications and repeated periodically to ensure serum uric acid levels are maintaining at appropriate levels while on therapy. The target serum uric acid for those with a diagnosis of gout is less than 6 mg/dL and less than 5 mg/dL for persons with tophaceous gout.[34] Urate-lowering medications should be adjusted accordingly to obtain these target serum uric acid levels.

VASCULITIS

The vasculitides are a family of conditions defined by inflammatory changes occurring in blood vessels. The numerous types of vasculitis are classified based on the size of the vessel affected: small, medium, or large.[35] Vasculitis may be a primary condition or occur secondary to another cause. These inflammatory vascular changes may lead to ischemic or necrotic complications. For the purposes of this discussion of pertinent laboratory tests associated with the vasculitides, only PMR, GCA, and granulomatosis with polyangiitis (GPA) are discussed in this article. GPA was formerly known as Wegener's granulomatosis.

Polymyalgia Rheumatica and Giant Cell Arteritis

PMR is an inflammatory condition affecting persons over the age of 50, with a peak incidence between the ages of 70 and 80 years.[36] PMR presents with aching and morning stiffness in proximal locations of the body, such as the shoulders, neck, and hips. GCA is the most common systemic vasculitis.[37] GCA is a large and medium vessel vasculitis that may affect the aorta and the cranial branches off the aortic arch. The most feared symptom of GCA is blindness. Fifteen percent of persons with PMR are estimated to have GCA, whereas 40% to 50% of persons with primarily GCA symptoms will have PMR.[38] The erythrocyte sedimentation rate (ESR) and C-reactive protein (CRP) are laboratory tests that can aid in diagnosing and monitoring PMR and GCA disease activity.

Erythrocyte sedimentation rate

The ESR is the rate at which red blood cells settle in a vertical tube and is felt to be a measure of acute phase reaction. The laboratory test is nonspecific because elevations in the ESR may be attributable to inflammation, infection, malignancy, tissue injury or ischemia, trauma, increased age, female gender, anemia, renal disease, obesity, and laboratory processing of sera. The ESR is elevated in PMR and GCA. At times, the ESR may exceed 100 mm/h, but an elevated sedimentation rate does not always correlate with disease activity. Some patients with PMR, estimated between 5% and 20%, may have an ESR of less than 40 mm/h[39-41]

C-reactive protein
CRP plays an integral part in the recognition and elimination of antigens in the function of the immune system. Elevations of CRP may occur, similar to the ESR, for inflammatory and infectious reasons and is therefore nonspecific, but helpful in diagnosing and monitoring inflammatory disease activity. Because both the ESR and CRP are nonspecific laboratory tests, when used together they aid a health care provider in diagnosing and monitoring PMR and GCA.

Granulomatosis with polyangiitis
GPA is a small vessel vasculitis that may be associated with the following signs and symptoms as per the ACR 1990 Classification Criteria.[42]

- Nasal or oral inflammation with painful or painless oral ulcers and purulent or bloody nasal discharge.
- Abnormal chest radiograph with nodules, fixed infiltrates, or cavities.
- Abnormal urinary sediment that manifests as microscopic hematuria with or without red cell casts.
- Granulomatous inflammation on biopsy of an artery or perivascular area.

Antineutrophil cytoplasmic antibodies (ANCA) is the laboratory test most often associated with GPA.

Antineutrophil cytoplasmic antibodies
ANCA is found in approximately 92% of patients with GPA[43] and should be performed on any patient suspected of having a systemic vasculitide. ANCA results are reported either as antibodies to myeloperoxidase, protease 3, or atypical, with GPA most commonly associated with the protease 3-ANCA. Over time, it has been suggested that increasing or decreasing ANCA results may be a means for measuring vasculitic disease activity. This notion remains controversial and unproven,[44] and thus the ANCA result should not solely be used to make treatment or follow-up decisions. As with other laboratory test results, including the ANCA results as a part of the decision-making process is recommended.

INFLAMMATORY MYOPATHIES

Inflammatory myopathies are characterized by proximal skeletal muscle weakness and muscle inflammation. The most commonly known inflammatory myopathies are polymyositis and dermatomyositis. The prevalence of polymyositis and dermatomyositis combined is estimated at 21.5 per 100,000.[45] Creatinine kinase and aldolase are muscle enzyme measures that can be used initially when screening for suspicion of an inflammatory myopathy and may be used to monitor response to treatment over time. Additionally, when elevated liver enzymes such as aspartate aminotransferase and alanine aminotransferase are noted to be increased, health care providers considering these results must consider the possibility of a muscle contribution to the elevated liver enzymes.

Diagnostic Autoantibodies in Inflammatory Myopathies

Autoantibodies are helpful from both a diagnostic and a prognostic perspective when treating a person with inflammatory myopathy. Three autoantibodies are briefly mentioned herein. Antisynthetase antibodies, the most common being anti–Jo-1, can be associated with idiopathic inflammatory myopathies. Antisynthetase antibodies can clinically be associated with interstitial lung disease, Raynaud phenomenon, arthritis, and mechanic's hands. Anti–signal recognition particle antibodies are almost exclusively found in polymyositis. Anti–signal recognition particle is often associated with aggressive and severe muscle disease. Anti–Mi-2 antibodies most commonly occur in dermatomyositis. These antibodies often manifest clinically with the acute onset of disease and with the shawl or V sign, a dermatologic feature of dermatomyositis.

FIBROMYALGIA

Although there is no single diagnostic test to confirm or monitor disease activity in fibromyalgia, laboratory studies, when appropriately ordered, do have a role in ruling out other conditions that may mimic fibromyalgia. Systemic review laboratory studies such as blood counts and chemistries, thyroid function laboratory tests, muscle enzyme laboratory tests, acute phase reactants, and appropriate autoantibodies like RF, CCP, and ANA might be considered. The decision to order specific laboratory tests should be determined by a person's signs, symptoms, and history in the appropriate clinical setting.

OSTEOARTHRITIS

Although OA is the most common form of arthritis globally, there are no current diagnostic laboratory tests for OA. OA treatments such as nonsteroidal antiinflammatory medications the require monitoring of renal and to a lesser extent hepatic function with their chronic use.

LABORATORY MONITORING FOR DISEASE TREATMENT

The treatment of rheumatic disease often requires the use of powerful immunosuppressants. These treatments require laboratory screening before their use and ongoing monitoring when a patient is being treated with immunosuppressants. The ACR has provided guidelines for laboratory monitoring when medications are used.[46–48] Biologics and small molecule medications also require predrug screening laboratory tests and ongoing laboratory monitoring.[49] **Tables 3** and **4** summarize these recommendations.

Table 3
Recommended laboratory evaluation for starting, resuming or significant dose increase for selected medications

Therapeutic Agents	CBC	Transaminases	Creatinine	Other
HCQ	X	X	X	Eye examination
LEF	X	X	X	Hepatitis serologies if patient is at risk
MTX	X	X	X	Hepatitis serologies if patient is at risk
Minocycline	X	X	X	
SSZ	X	X	X	
Biologics	X	X	X	

Abbreviations: CBC, complete blood count; HCQ, hydroxychloroquine; LEF, leflunomide; MTX, methotrexate; SSZ, sulfasalazine.

Adapted from Saag KG, Teng GG, Patkar NM, et al. American College of Rheumatology 2008 recommendations for the use of nonbiologic and biologic disease-modifying antirheumatic drugs in rheumatoid arthritis. Arthritis Rheum 2008;59:762–84.

Table 4
Recommended optimal laboratory follow-up monitoring (complete blood count, kidney and liver function) for selected medications

Therapeutic Agent	<3 mo	3-6 mo	>6 mo
HCQ	None after baseline	None	None
LEF	2–4 wk	6–12 wk	12 wk
MTX	2–4 wk	6–12 wk	12 wk
Minocycline	None after baseline	None	None
SSZ	2–4 wk	6–12 wk	12 wk

Abbreviations: HCQ, hydroxychloroquine; LEF, leflunomide; MTX, methotrexate; SSZ, sulfasalazine.
Adapted from Saag KG, Teng GG, Patkar NM, et al. American College of Rheumatology 2008 recommendations for the use of nonbiologic and biologic disease-modifying antirheumatic drugs in rheumatoid arthritis. Arthritis Rheum 2008;59:762–84.

SUMMARY

Diagnosing rheumatic disease can be challenging owing to the complex nature of these inflammatory, multi-system conditions. Appropriately selected laboratory tests can aid health care providers when diagnosing and monitoring persons with rheumatic disease. Being able to confidently explain laboratory indications and results to patients is a desired skill.

REFERENCES

1. Smith BJ, Bolster MB, Slusher B, et al. Core curriculum to facilitate the expansion of a rheumatology practice to include nurse practitioners and physician assistants. Arthritis Care Res 2018;70(5):672–8.
2. Barra L, Pope JE, Orav JE, et al. Prognosis of seronegative patients in a large prospective cohort of patients with early inflammatory arthritis. J Rheumatol 2014;41:2361–9.
3. Sokka T, Kautiainen H, Pincus T, et al. Disparities in rheumatoid arthritis disease activity according to gross domestic product in 25 countries in the QUEST-RA database. Ann Rheum Dis 2009;68:1666–72.
4. Chikkalingaiah KBM. Seronegative lupus membranous nephropathy. Int J Case Rep Imag 2016;7(10):624–7.
5. Cairns SA, Acheson EJ, Corbett CL, et al. The delayed appearance of an antinuclear factor and the diagnosis of systemic lupus erythematosus in glomerulonephritis. Postgrad Med J 1979;55(648):723–7.
6. Enriquez JL, Rajaraman S, Kalia A, et al. Isolated antinuclear antibody-negative lupus nephropathy in young children. Child Nephrol Urol 1988-1989;9(6):340–6.
7. Baskin E, Agras PI, Menekse N, et al. Full-house nephropathy in a patient with negative serology for lupus. Rheumatol Int 2007;27(3):281–4.
8. Bohan A. Seronegative systemic lupus erythematosus. J Rheumatol 1979;6(5):534–40.
9. Reichlin M. ANA negative systemic lupus erythematosus sera revisited serologically. Lupus 2000;9(2):116–9.
10. Arbuckle MR, McClain MT, Rubertone MV, et al. Development of autoantibodies before the clinical onset of systemic lupus erythematosus. N Engl J Med 2003;349:1526–33.

11. Heinlen LD, McClain MT, Merrill J, et al. Clinical criteria for systemic lupus erythematosus precede diagnosis, and associated autoantibodies are present before clinical symptoms. Arthritis Rheum 2007;56:2344–51.

12. Nielen MM, van Schaardenburg D, Reesink HW, et al. Specific autoantibodies precede the symptoms of rheumatoid arthritis: a study of serial measurements in blood donors. Arthritis Rheum 2004;50:380–6.

13. Waaler E. On the occurrence of a factor in human serum activating the specific agglutination of sheep corpuscles. APMIS 2007;115:422–38.

14. Hobbs K. Laboratory evaluation. In: West SG, editor. Rheumatology secrets. 3rd edition. Philadelphia: Elsevier Mosby; 2015. p. 48–57.

15. Whiting PF, Smidt N, Sterne JA, et al. Systematic review: accuracy of anti-citrullinated peptide antibodies to diagnosing rheumatoid arthritis. Ann Intern Med 2010;152(7):456.

16. Hargraves MM. Discovery of the LE cell and its morphology. Mayo Clin Proc 1969;44:579–99.

17. American College of Rheumatology. Methodology of testing for antinuclear antibodies. American College of Rheumatology. 2016. Available at: https://www.rheumatology.org/Portals/0/Files/Methodology%20of%20Testing%20Antinuclear%20Antibodies%20Position%20Statement.pdf. Accessed October 15 2018.

18. Avaniss-Aghajani E, Berzon S, Sarkissian A. Clinical value of multiplexed bead based immunoassays for detection of autoantibodies to nuclear antigens. Clin Vaccine Immunol 2007;14:505–9.

19. Bernardini S, Infantino M, Bellincampi L, et al. Screening of antinuclear antibodies: comparison between enzyme immunoassay based on nuclear homogenates, purified or recombinant antigens and immunofluorescence assay. Clin Chem Lab Med 2004;42:1155–60.

20. Biagini RE, Parks CG, Smith JP, et al. Analytical performance of the AtheNA Multi-Lyte ANA II assay in sera from lupus patients with multiple positive ANAs. Anal Bioanal Chem 2004;388:613–8.

21. Bonilla E, Francis L, Allam F, et al. Immunofluorescence microscopy is superior to fluorescent beads for detection of antinuclear antibody reactivity in systemic lupus erythematosus patients. Clin Immunol 2007;124:18–21.

22. Tan EM, Feltkamp TE, Smolen JS, et al. Range of antinuclear antibodies in "healthy" individuals. Arthritis Rheum 1997;40:1601–11.

23. Mahler M, Ngo JT, Schulte-Pelkum J, et al. Limited reliability of the indirect immunofluorescence technique for the detection of anti-Rib-P antibodies. Arthritis Res Ther 2008;10:R131.

24. Barada FA Jr, Andrews BS, Davis JS 4th, et al. Antibodies to Sm in patients with systemic lupus erythematosus. Correlation of Sm antibody titers with disease activity and other laboratory parameters. Arthritis Rheum 1981;24(10):1236–44.

25. Beaufils M, Kouki F, Mignon F, et al. Clinical significance of anti-Sm antibodies in systemic lupus erythematosus. Am J Med 1983;74(2):201–5.

26. Phan TG, Wong RC, Adelstein S. Autoantibodies to extractable nuclear antigens: making detection and interpretation more meaningful. Clin Diagn Lab Immunol 2002;9(1):1–7.

27. Yazdany J, Schmajuk G, Robbins M, et al. Choosing wisely: The American College of Rheumatology's top 5 list of things physicians and patients should question. Arthritis Care Res 2013;65:329–39.

28. Kavanaugh A, Tomar R, Reveille J, et al. Guidelines for clinical use of the antinuclear antibody test and tests for specific autoantibodies to nuclear antigens. American College of Pathologists. Arch Pathol Lab Med 2000;124(1):71–81.

29. Mathieu A, Paladini F, Vacca A, et al. The interplay between the geographic distribution of HLA-B27 alleles and their role in infectious and autoimmune diseases: a unifying hypothesis. Autoimmun Rev 2009;8(5):420–5.
30. Bakland G, Nossent HC. Epidemiology of spondyloarthritis: a review. Curr Rheumatol Rep 2013;15(9):351–7.
31. Kiltz U, Baraliakos X, Karakostas P, et al. Do patients with non-radiographic axial spondylarthritis differ from patients with ankylosing spondylitis? Arthritis Care Res 2012;64(9):1415–22.
32. Sieper J, van der Heijde D. Review: nonradiographic axial spondyloarthritis: new definition of an old disease? Arthritis Rheum 2013;65(3):543–51.
33. Janson RW. Ankylosing spondylitis. In: West SG, editor. Rheumatology secrets. 3rd edition. Philadelphia: Elsevier Mosby; 2015. p. 261–7.
34. Khanna D, Khanna P, Neogi T, et al. 2012 American College of Rheumatology guidelines for management of Gout. Part 1: systematic nonpharmacologic and pharmacologic therapeutic approaches to hyperuricemia. Arthritis Care Res 2012;64:1431–46.
35. Jennette JC, Falk RJ, Bacon PA, et al. 2012 revised International Chapel Hill consensus conference nomenclature of vasculitides. Arthritis Rheum 2013;65(1):1–11.
36. Salvarani C, Gabriel SE, O'Fallon WM, et al. Epidemiology of polymyalgia rheumatica in Olmstead County Minnesota, 1970-1991. Arthritis Rheum 1995;38(3):369–73.
37. Gonzalez-Gay MA, Garcia-Porrua C. Systemic vasculitis in adults in northwestern Spain, 1988-1997. Clinical and epidemiologic aspects. Medicine 1999;78(5):292–308.
38. Gonzalez-Gay MA, Barros S, Lopez-Diaz MJ, et al. Giant cell arteritis: disease patterns of clinical presentation in a series of 240 patients. Medicine 2005;84(5):269–76.
39. Helfgott SM, Kieval RI. Polymyalgia Rheumatica in patients with normal erythrocyte sedimentation rate. Arthritis Rheum 1996;39(2):304–7.
40. Gonzalez-Gay MA, Rodriguez-Valverde V, Blanco R, et al. Polymyalgia rheumatica without significantly increased erythrocyte sedimentation rate. A more benign syndrome. Arch Intern Med 1997;157(3):317–20.
41. Proven A, Gabriel SE, O'Fallon WM, et al. Polymyalgia rheumatica with low erythrocyte sedimentation rate at diagnosis. J Rheumatol 1999;26(6):1333–7.
42. Leavitt RY, Facui AS, Bloch DA, et al. The American College of Rheumatology 1990 criteria for the classification of Wegener's granulomatosis. Arthritis Rheum 1990;33(8):1101–7.
43. Finkielman JD, Lee AS, Hummel AM, et al, WGET Research Group. ANCA are detectable in nearly all patients with active severe Wegener's granulomatosis. Am J Med 2007;120(7):643.e9-14.
44. Tomasson G, Grayson PC, Mahr AD, et al. Value of ANCA measurements during remission to predict a relapse of ANCA-associated vasculitis-a meta-analysis. Rheumatology (Oxford) 2012;51(1):100–9.
45. Bernatsky S, Joshep L, Pineau CA, et al. Estimating the prevalence of polymyositis and dermatomyositis from administrative data: age, sex, and regional differences. Ann Rheum Dis 2009;68(7):1192–6.
46. Singh JA, Saag KG, Bridges SL Jr, et al. 2015 American College of Rheumatology guideline for the treatment of rheumatoid arthritis. Arthritis Rheum 2016;68(1):1–26.

47. Singh JA, Furst DE, Bharat A, et al. 2012 update of the 2008 American College of Rheumatology recommendations for the use of disease-modifying antirheumatic drugs and biologic agents in the treatment of rheumatoid arthritis. Arthritis Care Res 2012;64(5):625–39.
48. Saag KG, Teng GG, Patkar NM, et al. American College of Rheumatology 2008 recommendations for the use of non biologic and biologic disease-modifying antirheumatic drugs in rheumatoid arthritis. Arthritis Rheum 2008;59(6):762–84.
49. Smith BJ, Nuccio BC, Graves KY, et al. Screening and work-up requirements prior to beginning biologic medications for dermatologic and rheumatic diseases. J Am Acad Physician Assist 2018;31(6):23–8.

Update in the Molecular Diagnostics of Sexually Transmitted Infections

Robert Paxton, PA-C, MPAS[a],*, Erik Munson, PhD, D(ABMM)[b],
Kathleen Barta, PA-C, MPAS[c]

KEYWORDS

- STI • NAAT • Molecular testing • *Neisseria gonorrhoeae* • *Chlamydia trachomatis*
- *Mycoplasma genitalium* • *Trichomonas vaginalis*

KEY POINTS

- Sexually transmitted infections (STIs) are common in the United States and the diagnosis may not be considered without thorough evaluation of risk factors/historical considerations.
- Most nonulcerative STIs are asymptomatic/minimally symptomatic in both men and women.
- Historically, the diagnosis of STIs has suffered from suboptimal sensitivity and specificity. Nucleic acid amplification testing (NAAT) has revolutionized the diagnosis of many nonulcerative STIs.
- The incidence of *Mycoplasma genitalium* is starting to be more fully appreciated due to the diagnostic accuracy of NAAT.

INTRODUCTION

In this article, we review and assess the use of molecular assays in diagnosing some of the most common bacterial sexually transmitted infections (STIs) in the United States: *Neisseria gonorrhoeae, Chlamydia trachomatis, Mycoplasma genitalium,* and *Trichomonas vaginalis*. Use of molecular testing, using specific DNA or RNA sequences in urine and or other sources, has rapidly increased and improved over the past 10 years.

According to the Centers for Disease Control and Prevention, the performance of nucleic acid amplification tests (NAATs) with respect to overall sensitivity,

Disclosure Statement: E. Munson has received research support from Hologic, Incorporated.
[a] Department of Physician Assistant Studies, College of Health Sciences, Marquette University, PO Box 1881, Milwaukee, WI 53201-1881, USA; [b] Department of Clinical Laboratory Science, College of Health Sciences, Marquette University, PO Box 1881, Milwaukee, WI 53201-1881, USA; [c] Infectious Disease Specialists of Southeastern Wisconsin, Brookfield, WI 53005, USA
* Corresponding author.
E-mail address: Robert.paxton@marquette.edu

Physician Assist Clin 4 (2019) 501–518
https://doi.org/10.1016/j.cpha.2019.02.003
2405-7991/19/© 2019 Elsevier Inc. All rights reserved.

physicianassistant.theclinics.com

specificity, and ease of specimen transport is better than that of any other testing method available for the diagnosis of chlamydial and gonococcal infections. NAAT amplify and detect nucleic acid sequences that are organism specific. Because NAAT do not require viable organisms for diagnosis, a minimal specimen of target DNA or RNA is needed. This has resulted in higher sensitivity, enabling less invasive testing procedures, such as first-catch urine or vaginal swab.

Diagnosis of *M genitalium* traditionally has been difficult. NAAT is now the preferred technique, and can be used on urethral, vaginal, and cervical swabs, and on urine specimens. For many years, *T vaginalis* infections have been diagnosed with wet-mount microscopic examination and culture. However, NAAT, although not as available as the wet-mount, when done on urine and vaginal swabs has shown improved sensitivity and specificity over previous testing methods.

Although culture was previously the preferred method for most STI testing, it can be expensive, difficult to standardize, challenging to maintain viability of organisms during transport, and has low sensitivity.[1] Since 2002, improvement in molecular assay testing has resulted in faster and easier implementation and expansion of screening for many STIs. In turn, this allows clinicians to identify infections at an earlier stage, select treatments, prevent further transmission, and reduce inappropriate antibiotic prescribing.

OVERVIEW OF MOLECULAR DIAGNOSTICS
Nucleic Acid Hybridization Versus Nucleic Acid Amplification

Laboratory options for adjunctive diagnosis of nonulcerative STIs that are discussed within this report include microscopy, culture, serology, antigen detection, and molecular diagnostics. While reviewing literature pertinent to molecular-based options, one must be cognizant of fundamental delineations between nucleic acid hybridization assays and NAAT. Nucleic acid hybridization uses oligonucleotide sequences (often linked to radiographic, colorimetric, or fluorescent reporters) that are designed to anneal to complementary nucleic acid sequences from the organism of interest; as such, target nucleic acid is detected in direct fashion. In contrast, NAAT uses 2 stages of oligonucleotide reactions. The first involves amplification of target nucleic acid by specific oligonucleotide annealing or priming; the second uses an additional set of complementary reporter-linked oligonucleotide probes to allow for detection of amplified target.

Rapid turnaround time can be realized because traditional target amplification is not incorporated into nucleic acid hybridization. Selected assays have been adapted to semiautomated platforms to enhance laboratory or point-of-care workflow. However, deficiencies in analytical sensitivity exist within clinical nucleic acid hybridization assays, largely as a function of organism burden within a specimen. As one example (peripheral to the nonulcerative STI agents described in this report), Briselden and Hillier[2] evaluated commercial nucleic acid hybridization for direct detection of *Gardnerella vaginalis*–specific nucleic acid from vaginal swabs compared with a culture reference. Positive results were yielded by 95% of specimens containing greater than 5×10^5 colony-forming units of *G vaginalis*/mL. In contrast, 43% of specimens harboring $\leq 5 \times 10^5$ colony-forming units of *G vaginalis*/mL yielded a positive nucleic acid hybridization result. Because of analytical sensitivity issues inherent to nucleic acid hybridization, this method is reserved for scenarios (both clinical and laboratory culture confirmation) in which high nucleic acid target burden is anticipated.[3]

Basic Tenets and Comparisons of DNA Amplification and RNA Amplification

In a simplistic sense, NAAT modalities can be classified into those using DNA amplification and those using RNA amplification. Dating back 30 years, basic research data exist comparing the efficiency of DNA and RNA amplification techniques. The seminal report of the DNA amplification technique polymerase chain reaction[4] noted a 10^6-fold rate of DNA amplification in 3 to 4 hours. In contrast, an RNA amplification technique known as transcription-mediated amplification increased RNA target at a 10^9-fold rate within 2 hours.[5]

For nearly 15 years, it has been postulated that analogous differences exist between STI testing formats of DNA and RNA amplification.[6] Chernesky and colleagues[7] prepared mock clinical swab specimens containing propagated C trachomatis elementary bodies and showed that analytical sensitivity of RNA amplification was 10-fold to 1000-fold greater than 2 commercial DNA amplification assays. RNA amplification furthermore exhibited 100-fold greater sensitivity than the same comparators with mock urine specimens. This in vitro concept was further validated with data published by Ikeda-Dantsuji and colleagues[8] in which standardized quantities of C trachomatis elementary bodies were distributed into mock clinical specimens. Subsequent dilution series demonstrated commercial RNA amplification sensitivity being 1000-fold greater than commercial DNA amplification. Wood and colleagues[9] demonstrated a lower limit of detection for N gonorrhoeae via RNA amplification (10^2 colony-forming units/mL) than that rendered by DNA amplification modalities ($\geq 10^3$ colony-forming units/mL).

Nye and colleagues[10] assessed microscopic direct detection, culture, and NAAT for the detection of T vaginalis. When using a reference standard composed of positive direct detection or culture result from women, amplification methods yielded sensitivity values (depending on specimen source) ranging from 91.3% to 98.6% (DNA amplification) and 98.6% (RNA amplification), in comparison to the 95.7% value for T vaginalis culture. Specificity values for DNA and RNA amplification testing were 97.8% to 98.2% and 92.5% to 96.0%, respectively, based on the aforementioned reference standard. Alternatively, when the reference standard was a composite of any positive test result (including traditional testing methods and either amplification assay), sensitivity of RNA amplification on female urine, endocervical, and vaginal specimens was 87.5%, 89.8%, and 96.6%, respectively. Analogous values derived from polymerase chain reaction (PCR) were 76.1%, 80.9%, and 83.0%. The same trend was noted during analysis of first-void male urine and urethral swab specimens. Sensitivity of RNA amplification ranged from 73.8% (urine) to 95.2% (urethral swab) when using the reference standard inclusive of all molecular tests. Corresponding sensitivity data from DNA amplification were 47.6% and 54.8%, respectively. Health professionals are advised to consider the reference standard used in published assessments of diagnostic assays. Moreover, analogous to other bacterial[11,12] and virus[13,14] systems in which new molecular reference standards have emerged, RNA amplification positions itself as an updated reference standard in the molecular detection of STI agents.

Beyond the robust cellular process of transcription by which up to 1000 RNA transcripts are synthesized from a single DNA template, one explanation for differences in clinical and analytical sensitivity between RNA and DNA amplification may lie in multiplicity of target nucleic acid. As one example, up to 10,000 copies of the C trachomatis ribosomal RNA target for a commercial RNA amplification modality are found per cell,[15] whereas C trachomatis cells contain approximately 10 copies of plasmid DNA target for one commercial DNA amplification assay. A second contributory factor may be related to endogenous inhibitors of NAAT. Substances noted to inhibit *C trachomatis* NAAT have included hemoglobin, low-pH cervical mucosa, β-chorionic gonadotropin, urine crystals, and urine nitrites.[16–18] Ikeda-Dantsuji and colleagues[8] additionally reported deleterious effects of increased concentrations of iron and phosphate on *C trachomatis* amplification testing. One first-generation RNA amplification assay revealed an 11.9% rate of amplification inhibition from 388 urine specimens.[16] However, incorporation of a target capture protocol (using magnetic-coupled organism-specific oligonucleotides) into a second-generation RNA amplification assay, with concomitant exposure to magnetic field, washing, and aspiration, has largely negated this inhibitory effect. One subsequent study[7] revealed inhibition rates of 0.3% and 1.3% to 1.7% from urine and female genital swab specimens, respectively, when using a second-generation RNA amplification assay using target capture.

Inhibitors endogenous to gastrointestinal specimens have been described.[19] Thus, the aforementioned factors (particularly the removal of endogenous inhibitors by oligonucleotide target capture) have not only facilitated screening of urogenital specimens but also allow for accurate screening of extragenital specimens from selected high-risk demographics by RNA amplification assays. As one example, Schachter and colleagues[20] reported 44.4% sensitivity of one commercial DNA amplification assay for detection of *N gonorrhoeae* from rectal specimens when compared with second-generation commercial RNA amplification. The investigators noted 60% sensitivity of commercial DNA amplification for detection of the agent from pharyngeal swabs. Commercial RNA amplification was also 12.4% and 14.8% more sensitive than a second format of DNA amplification in detection of *N gonorrhoeae* from pharyngeal and rectal sites, respectively. Ota and colleagues[21] reported 21.1% and 97.4% sensitivity of *C trachomatis* culture and 2 NAAT modalities, respectively, from rectal specimens from a high-risk demographic. A significant number of pharyngeal specimens yielded *C trachomatis* detection via NAAT in the face of a 0% culture-positive rate; 64.7% sensitivity of DNA amplification for detection of *C trachomatis* was demonstrated from rectal specimens when compared with second-generation RNA amplification.[21] The same study reported 33.3% DNA amplification sensitivity for pharyngeal *C trachomatis* detection. Furthermore, RNA amplification was 30% and 33% more sensitive than a second format of DNA amplification testing in detection of *C trachomatis* nucleic acid from rectal and pharyngeal sites, respectively.

In summary, NAAT modalities have become the reference method for laboratory detection of several STI agents. This particularly holds true for agents that are susceptible to specimen transport environments and those for which culture or direct microscopy techniques lack analytical sensitivity. Not all NAAT are created equal; RNA amplification assays have increased analytical sensitivity when compared with DNA amplification modalities. At the same time, clinicians must be cognizant of FDA-cleared indications for diagnostic assays (**Table 1**) provided by their local laboratory. Moreover, laboratories possessing significant resources and technical expertise have the opportunity to add laboratory-developed tests or laboratory-modified assays (eg, extra-urogenital specimen sources) onto testing menus.[22,23]

PATHOGENS
Neisseria gonorrhoeae

Gonorrhea, caused by the bacterium *N gonorrhoeae*, is the second most reported STI in the United States.[24] *N gonorrhoeae* infection is most commonly found in the mucus membranes of the reproductive tract in both men and women, but also may cause infection in the pharynx, rectum, skin, heart valves, and joints. Rarely it can

Table 1
Commercial molecular diagnostic testing options available in the United States and cleared by the Food and Drug Administration (FDA) for *Neisseria gonorrhoeae*, *Chlamydia trachomatis*, and *Trichomonas vaginalis*

General Format	Method	Distributor	Assay	FDA-Cleared Indications	Notes
Detection of *N gonorrhoeae* and/or *C trachomatis*-specific nucleic acid					
Nucleic acid hybridization	Hybrid capture	Digene Corporation	*digene* HC2 CT/GC[a] DNA Test (microplate platform)	Endocervical swab Endocervical brush	Symptomatic or asymptomatic patients; positive result requires additional assay performance
		Digene Corporation	*digene* HC2 GC-ID DNA Test (microplate platform)	Endocervical swab Endocervical brush	Symptomatic or asymptomatic patients; test is required follow-up to *digene* HC2 CT/GC DNA Test yielding positive result
		Digene Corporation	*digene* HC2 CT-ID DNA Test (microplate platform)	Endocervical swab Endocervical brush	Symptomatic or asymptomatic patients; test is required follow-up to *digene* HC2 CT/GC DNA Test yielding positive result
DNA amplification	Polymerase chain reaction	Abbott Molecular Incorporated	Abbott RealTime CT/NG[a] (Abbott *m2000* platform)	Endocervical swab Vaginal swab Urethral swab Patient-collected vaginal swab Female urine Male urine	Symptomatic or asymptomatic patients (with exception of endocervical and urethral swabs only indicated on symptomatic patients)
		BD Diagnostic Systems	BD MAX CT/GC/TV[a] assay (BD MAX platform)	Endocervical swab Patient-collected vaginal swab Female urine Male urine	Symptomatic or asymptomatic patients
		Cepheid	Xpert CT/NG[a] (GeneXpert Instrument platform)	Endocervical swab Patient-collected vaginal swab Female urine Male urine	Symptomatic or asymptomatic patients

(continued on next page)

Table 1
(continued)

General Format	Method	Distributor	Assay	FDA-Cleared Indications	Notes
		Roche Diagnostics Corporation	AMPLICOR CT/NG[a] Test	Endocervical swab Urethral swab Male urine	Symptomatic or asymptomatic patients (with exception of urethral swab only indicated on symptomatic patients)
		Roche Molecular Systems, Incorporated	cobas CT/NG[a] v2.0 Test (cobas 4800 platform)	Endocervical swab Vaginal swab PreservCyt collection Patient-collected vaginal swab Female urine Male urine	Symptomatic or asymptomatic patients
		Roche Molecular Systems, Incorporated	cobas CT/NG[a] (cobas 6800/8800 platform)	Endocervical swab Vaginal swab PreservCyt collection Patient-collected vaginal swab Female urine Male urine	Symptomatic or asymptomatic patients
	Strand displacement amplification	Becton, Dickinson and Company	BD ProbeTec *Neisseria gonorrhoeae* (GC) Q[x] Amplified DNA Assay (BD Viper or Viper LT platforms)	Endocervical swab Urethral swab PreservCyt, SurePath collection Patient-collected vaginal swab Female urine Male urine	Symptomatic or asymptomatic patients
		Becton, Dickinson and Company	BD ProbeTec *Chlamydia trachomatis* (CT) Q[x] Amplified DNA Assay (BD Viper or Viper LT platforms)	Endocervical swab Urethral swab PreservCyt, SurePath collection Patient-collected vaginal swab Female urine Male urine	Symptomatic or asymptomatic patients
		Becton, Dickinson and Company	BD ProbeTec ET *Chlamydia trachomatis* and *N gonorrhoeae*[a] Amplified DNA Assays (BD ProbeTec ET or Viper platforms)	Endocervical swab Urethral swab Female urine Male urine	Symptomatic or asymptomatic patients

RNA amplification	Transcription-mediated amplification	Hologic, Incorporated	Aptima Combo 2 Assay[a] (Panther platform)	Endocervical swab, Vaginal swab, Urethral swab, PreservCyt collection, Patient-collected vaginal swab, Female urine, Male urine	Symptomatic or asymptomatic patients
		Hologic, Incorporated	Aptima Combo 2 Assay[a] (Tigris or semiautomated platform)	Endocervical swab, Vaginal swab, Urethral swab, PreservCyt collection, Patient-collected vaginal swab, Female urine, Male urine	Symptomatic or asymptomatic patients (with exception of patient-collected vaginal swab only indicated on asymptomatic patients)
		Hologic, Incorporated	Aptima Neisseria gonorrhoeae Assay (Tigris or semiautomated platform)	Endocervical swab, Vaginal swab, Urethral swab, PreservCyt collection, Patient-collected vaginal swab, Female urine, Male urine	Symptomatic or asymptomatic patients (with exception of patient-collected vaginal swab only indicated on asymptomatic patients; with exception of urethral swab only indicated on symptomatic patients)
		Hologic, Incorporated	Aptima Chlamydia trachomatis Assay (Tigris or semiautomated platform)	Endocervical swab, Vaginal swab, Urethral swab, PreservCyt collection, Patient-collected vaginal swab, Female urine, Male urine	Symptomatic or asymptomatic patients (with exception of patient-collected vaginal swab only indicated on asymptomatic patients)

(continued on next page)

Table 1
(continued)

Detection of *M genitalium*-specific nucleic acid[b]

RNA amplification	Transcription-mediated amplification	Hologic, Incorporated	Aptima Mycoplasma genitalium Assay (Panther platform)	Endocervical swab Urethral swab Patient-collected vaginal swab Provider-collected vaginal swab Female urine Male urine Patient-collected penile swab	Symptomatic or asymptomatic patients

Detection of *T vaginalis*-specific nucleic acid

Nucleic acid hybridization	DNA probe	Becton, Dickinson and Company	Affirm VPIII Microbial Identification Test (manual platform)	Vaginal fluid specimens from patients with symptoms of vaginitis/vaginosis	Additional detection of *Candida albicans* and *Gardnerella vaginalis*

	Technology	Manufacturer	Assay (platform)	Specimen	Patient population
DNA amplification	Helicase-dependent amplification	Quidel Corporation	Solana *Trichomonas* Assay (Solana platform)	Vaginal swab, Female urine	Symptomatic or asymptomatic patients
	Polymerase chain reaction	BD Diagnostic Systems	BD MAX CT/GC/TV[a] assay (BD MAX platform)	Endocervical swab, Patient-collected vaginal swab, Female urine	Symptomatic or asymptomatic patients
		Cepheid	Xpert TV (GeneXpert Instrument platform)	Endocervical swab, Patient-collected vaginal swab, Female urine, Male urine	Symptomatic or asymptomatic patients
		GeneOhm Sciences (BD Diagnostics) Canada, Incorporated	BD MAX Vaginal Panel (BD MAX platform)	Vaginal swab	Symptomatic patients; additional detection of bacteria associated with bacterial vaginosis and *Candida* spp. associated with vulvovaginal candidiasis
	Strand displacement amplification	Becton, Dickinson and Company	BD ProbeTec *Trichomonas vaginalis* (TV) Q[x] Amplified DNA Assay (BD Viper platform)	Endocervical swab, Patient-collected vaginal swab, Female urine	Symptomatic or asymptomatic patients
RNA amplification	Transcription-mediated amplification	Hologic, Incorporated	Aptima *Trichomonas vaginalis* Assay (Panther platform)	Endocervical swab, Vaginal swab, PreservCyt collection	Symptomatic or asymptomatic patients
		Hologic, Incorporated	Aptima *Trichomonas vaginalis* Assay (Tigris platform)	Endocervical swab, Vaginal swab, Female urine, PreservCyt collection	Symptomatic or asymptomatic patients

Note: Patient-collected vaginal swabs are collected in a clinic setting (with instruction).

Abbreviations: CT, *chlamydia trachomatis*; GC, NG, *Neisseria gonorrhoeae*; TV, *Trichomonas vaginalis*.

[a] Simultaneous detection of *Neisseria gonorrhoeae*, *Chlamydia trachomatis*, and/or *Trichomonas vaginalis* nucleic acid from single primary specimen.

[b] No fewer than seven molecular diagnostic assays have been *Conformité Européenne* (CE)-marked for detection of *Mycoplasma genitalium*. Commercial availability of these assays may vary.

disseminate and cause blood stream infections, and skin and central nervous infections. Gonorrhea is transmitted through sexual contact with the penis, vagina, mouth, or anus from an infected partner.

The most common presentation of gonorrheal infection in men is acute urethritis, which typically presents with dysuria, and clear to mucoid penile discharge. Urethritis may also progress to epididymitis, with scrotal or testicular pain. Both men and women can develop proctitis, anal itching, rectal tenderness, and pain with bowel movements from anal infection.

The primary site of gonorrheal infection in women is the cervix, causing cervicitis. Patients may have vaginal discharge with clear to yellow drainage, vaginal bleeding, dysuria, or be completely asymptomatic. Left untreated, gonorrheal cervicitis may progress to the uterus or fallopian tubes causing pelvic inflammatory disease (PID), or tubo-ovarian abscess. PID in turn can lead to tubal scarring, causing infertility or ectopic pregnancy.[24]

Gonorrhea can be potentially diagnosed using NAAT on urine specimens from both men and women; endocervical or vaginal swabs for women; or from urethral swab for men.[24] Gonorrhea also can be cultivated from clinical specimens, as NAAT is not FDA-cleared for all potential clinical samples.[24]

Laboratory diagnosis of N gonorrhoeae is unique among nonulcerative STI in that direct detection methods provide clinical value. In one investigation, 94.8% of male N gonorrhoeae urethritis cases included a Gram stain indicating Gram-negative diplococci within neutrophils. This finding was not present in 92% of cases of nongonococcal urethritis (NGU).[25] Because N gonorrhoeae is a fastidious organism, optimal recovery of this pathogen is facilitated by media inoculation immediately after specimen collection. Several selective media with individualized supplements can cultivate N gonorrhoeae from primary clinical specimens, particularly from sources known to contain significant amounts of commensal flora.[26] In a nonlaboratory setting, inoculated media may incubate at room temperature in a commercial carbon dioxide–generating system during a transport interval without appreciable loss of organism viability.[27,28]

Swab transport systems typically represent a suitable means of preserving microbes before laboratory cultivation, yet this paradigm does not always apply to N gonorrhoeae. Arbique and colleagues[29] reported N gonorrhoeae recovery rates of 17% to 94% for 4 swab transport systems at 24 hours. This range dropped to 0.04% to 72% at 48 hours. In all systems tested, organism burden decreased by $\geq$80% within 6 hours of swab inoculation.[29] However, culture techniques procure viable organism for standardized antimicrobial susceptibility testing and subsequent antimicrobial resistance surveillance.

The ultimate benefit of NAAT for N gonorrhoeae may lie within the realm of specimen transport, as Livengood and Wrenn[30] demonstrated just a slight disparity in the rate of N gonorrhoeae detection from endocervical specimens by commercial DNA amplification (96.3%) versus N gonorrhoeae culture (92.6%). Similar to previous discussion in this review, studies have revealed increased analytical sensitivity of second-generation RNA amplification versus that of DNA amplification.[31,32] This paradigm extends to utilization of first-void urine as a primary specimen source in a number of FDA-cleared assays (see **Table 1**).

Chlamydia trachomatis

Urogenital C trachomatis infection is the most commonly reported bacterial STI in the United States, with the highest prevalence in patients younger than 24 years.[33] Most infections are asymptomatic for both men and women. Risk factors include younger age, multiple sexual partners, and prior chlamydial infection. Chlamydia is transmitted sexually but also can be spread perinatally from an untreated mother to her infant during childbirth, causing conjunctivitis or pneumonia in the infant.[33] Chlamydia infection is more prevalent in women, and disproportionately affects young non-Hispanic black women.[34]

Chlamydia is one of the most common causes of NGU in men. Men may have mild dysuria or penile discharge, but typically are asymptomatic. Men who have sex with men are at increased risk of anal infections and proctitis.

Cervicitis is the most common chlamydial infection in women, with symptoms ranging from pale to gray vaginal discharge, abnormal vaginal bleeding between periods or after intercourse, dyspareunia or dysuria. Most women are asymptomatic with chlamydia infections, and this may lead to delayed diagnosis and treatment. Lack of treatment may cause spread of infection to the upper reproductive tract, uterus, and fallopian tubes, causing PID, abdominal pain, and pelvic pain. Permanent damage to the uterus and fallopian tubes may result, causing chronic pelvic pain, infertility, and ectopic pregnancy. Annual screening of all sexually active women younger than 25 years is recommended, as is screening of older women at increased risk for infection, for example, those with multiple sex partners, new sex partners, or partners with known STI.[33]

Vaginal or endocervical swab is the best choice to screen for chlamydia infection in women; urine specimen is preferred in men. For pharyngeal and rectal chlamydia infections, culture is recommended, but can be compromised by suboptimal analytical sensitivity. However, cell culture for chlamydia is not available at most laboratories, consequently laboratory-modified NAAT is typically done on these specimens as well.[33]

For years, the accepted reference standard for C trachomatis detection was culture, including optimization in shell vials.[35] Culturing techniques in McCoy cell lines are complex and time-consuming, with the necessity for experienced laboratorians for accurate follow-up staining and microscopy. Early attempts at rapid detection of the organism included direct fluorescent antibody testing (DFA) and optical immunoassay (OIA). However, Boyadzhyan and colleagues[36] reported that C trachomatis culture and DFA and DFA detected ~25% and 0%, respectively, of specimens determined to be positive by NAAT. From a cohort of 1385 women, Swain and colleagues[37] reported sensitivity and specificity values of 73.6% and 99.9% (respectively) for DFA; 64.2% and 99.1% for OIA; 56.1% and 100% for culture; and 95.3% and 99.8% for NAAT.

In contrast to N gonorrhoeae NAAT, the inherent value of C trachomatis NAAT lies in analytical sensitivity. One early evaluation[38] reported 89.2% to 89.7% sensitivity of C trachomatis DNA amplification from female urine and endocervical specimens, respectively, with 88.6% to 90.3% sensitivity from male urethral and urine specimens. A second[31] demonstrated 94.2% C trachomatis RNA amplification sensitivity from endocervical specimens. Sensitivity of detection from female urine (94.7%) was markedly higher than DNA amplification. Specificity of RNA amplification was 97.6% for endocervical specimens and 98.9% for urine specimens.[31] In response to selected commercial DNA amplification assays demonstrating false-positive results in the context of N gonorrhoeae NAAT,[39–41] direct challenges of second-generation RNA amplification with nonpathogenic Neisseria spp and chlamydiae other than C trachomatis failed to result in amplification.[42]

Mycoplasma genitalium

M genitalium was first described in the 1980s in patients with NGU. The organism lacks a cell wall, which prevents utilization of the traditional Gram stain and it can take months to culture.[43] Given the issues with Gram stain and culture, the epidemiology of M *genitalium* did not start to be understood until the 1990s when PCR tests became available. This has led to a paucity of data about this STI. *M genitalium* is most commonly found in genitourinary and rectal tissues.[44] An estimated 1% to 2% of the general population is infected,[44] but *M genitalium* accounts for 15% to 20% of NGU cases, 20% to 25% of nonchlamydial NGU, and 30% of persistent/recurrent urethritis.[43]

The most common presentation of *M genitalium* infection in men is acute urethritis, as previously described. Asymptomatic infection is less common than in women.[45] The duration of asymptomatic infection is currently unknown.[44] Most *M genitalium* infections in women are asymptomatic as well.[44,45] Clinical presentation is most commonly cervicitis (as previously described), but it has also been associated with urethritis, PID, and adverse birth outcomes.[44–46]

In the clinical setting, the microbiological diagnosis of *M genitalium* has not been frequently performed due to a paucity of diagnostic options. In the research setting, M genitalium has been detected from urine, urethral, vaginal, or cervical swabs, and endometrial biopsies.[43] The optimal sample type continues to be researched. Recent European guidelines recommend first-void urine testing and/or vaginal swabs in women.[44,45]

However, culture techniques applied to specimens from either gender are limited by the fastidious nature of *M genitalium*.[47–49] Serologic diagnosis of this agent has met with difficulty[50–52] and is further complicated by antigenic variation exhibited by the bacterium[53,54] and immunogenic proteins resembling analogs found in *Mycoplasma pneumoniae*.[55]

M genitalium NAAT development represents a highly evolving field.[56] One RNA amplification assay (**Table 1**) received FDA clearance in January 2019. The assay is indicated for testing of both asymptomatic and symptomatic individuals using endocervical, urethral, vaginal (both patient- and provider-collected), and patient-collected penile swabs, as well as female and male first-void urine specimens. In one RNA amplification investigation of first-void male urine specimens in a high-prevalence population, *M genitalium* detection rates were similar to *C trachomatis*.[57] Detection rates of *M genitalium* from women exceeded *T vaginalis* and *C trachomatis* in the same population.[58] Outpatient obstetric clinics demonstrated particularly high rates of *M genitalium* detection and additional data espouse first-void urine as a means of screening women for *M genitalium*. Chernesky and colleagues[59] reported increased *M genitalium* detection from self-collected penile swabs compared with first-void urine. Management of macrolide-resistant *M genitalium* in the clinical setting has prompted research efforts into molecular-based assays for simultaneous detection of *M genitalium*–specific nucleic acid and macrolide resistance determinants.[60,61]

Trichomonas vaginalis

T vaginalis is a flagellated protozoan that is known to infect only humans. Sexual activity is the predominate mode of transmission. Epidemiologically, trichomoniasis is more evenly spread among sexually active women of all ages. The overall prevalence ranges from 3% to 13% but depends on the population studied.[62] *T vaginalis* commonly coexist with the organisms that cause bacterial vaginosis as well as other STIs, particularly gonorrhea.[62] It is the most prevalent nonviral STI in the United States.[43] *T vaginalis* principally infects reproductive tissue, like other previously mentioned STIs.

Trichomanias in men is frequently asymptomatic with rapid spontaneous resolution. If symptomatic, trichomoniasis usually presents with urethritis, which may progress to epididymitis or prostatitis.[43] As with men, women are frequently asymptomatic. The most common presentation is vaginitis, which may present with malodorous discharge, pruritis, dyspareunia, and dysuria. As with other previously described STIs, trichomoniasis may also present as urethritis.

Trichomoniasis can be diagnosed from a variety of clinical samples depending on the test performed. Common specimens include vaginal or endocervical swabs, or urine samples in women. Men are most frequently sampled with first-void urine or urethral swab specimens.[43]

Trichomoniasis prevalence rates are likely underestimated.[63] Wet mount is a common means of *T vaginalis* detection. Advantages of this method include cost and predictive value of motile parasite observation,[64] resulting in rapid turnaround time. Sensitivity has ranged from 58% to 86%.[65–68] *T vaginalis* culture has traditionally served as a reference method. However, limitations include turnaround time[69] and clinical laboratories being less likely to maintain cell culture capacity. Levi and colleagues[70] reported 82.4% sensitivity of a commercial culture system. Approximately 80% of positive cultures were detectable within 24 hours of inoculation.

Antigen testing can provide a point-of-care *T vaginalis* assessment. Commercial antigen test sensitivity and specificity was reported at 89.6% and 97.5%, respectively, compared with a composite wet mount/culture standard.[71] In this study, discrepancies in wet mount and antigen test performance were noted between symptomatic and asymptomatic patients. However, recent data have demonstrated that *T vaginalis* antigen testing yields greater accuracy in high-prevalence populations, irrespective of patient symptoms.[72]

Sensitivity values of the aforementioned methods, in addition to methods involving nucleic acid hybridization, have decreased with the emergence of NAAT.[63] Within a population of 5% *T vaginalis* prevalence, Andrea and Chapin[73] reported 63.4% sensitivity of commercial nucleic acid hybridization compared with a NAAT reference; 46.3% sensitivity of nucleic acid hybridization compared with NAAT was observed in a population exhibiting 16.9% *T vaginalis* prevalence.[74] Not only does NAAT provide high accuracy of testing, but it also lends new insight into the epidemiology of trichomoniasis.[75]

SUMMARY

STIs are common in the United States, and some unfortunately are on the rise, especially in certain geographic areas and patient populations. The diagnosis has historically been challenging because many of these diseases are asymptomatic/minimally symptomatic and laboratory diagnosis frequently suffers from less than optimal sensitivity and specificity. Concurrent infection with multiple STIs is also not uncommon. One new example of how important NAAT diagnostics will prove to be is in the diagnosis of *M genitalium*, which is being labeled as a potential new superbug.[76] Given the new molecular diagnostics now available, a new approach to STI diagnosis is on the horizon.

REFERENCES

1. Papp JR, Schachter J, Gaydos CA, et al. Recommendations for the laboratory-based detection of *Chlamydia trachomatis* and *Neisseria gonorrhoeae* – 2014. MMWR Recomm Rep 2014;63(RR02):1–19.
2. Briselden AM, Hillier SH. Evaluation of Affirm VP microbial identification test for *Gardnerella vaginalis* and *Trichomonas vaginalis*. J Clin Microbiol 1994;32:148–52.
3. Nolte FS. Molecular microbiology. In: Jorgensen JH, Pfaller MA, Carroll KC, et al, editors. Manual of clinical microbiology. 11th edition. Washington, DC: ASM Press; 2015. p. 54–90.

4. Saiki RK, Gelfand DH, Stoffel S, et al. Primer-directed enzymatic amplification of DNA with a thermostable DNA polymerase. Science 1988;239:487–91.

5. Compton J. Nucleic acid sequence-based amplification. Nature 1991;350:91–2.

6. Schachter J, Hook EW, Martin DH, et al. Confirming positive results of nucleic acid amplification tests (NAATs) for *Chlamydia trachomatis*: all NAATs are not created equal. J Clin Microbiol 2005;43:1372–3.

7. Chernesky M, Jang D, Luinstra K, et al. High analytical sensitivity and low rates of inhibition may contribute to detection of *Chlamydia trachomatis* in significantly more women by the APTIMA Combo 2 assay. J Clin Microbiol 2006;44:400–5.

8. Ikeda-Dantsuji Y, Konomi I, Nagayama A. *In vitro* assessment of the APTIMA Combo 2 assay for the detection of *Chlamydia trachomatis* using highly purified elementary bodies. J Med Microbiol 2005;54:357–60.

9. Wood BJ, Rizzo-Price P, Holden J, et al. The microbicide tenofovir does not inhibit nucleic acid amplification tests for detection of *Chlamydia trachomatis* and *Neisseria gonorrhoeae* in urine samples. J Clin Microbiol 2008;46:763–5.

10. Nye MB, Schwebke JR, Body BA. Comparison of APTIMA *Trichomonas vaginalis* transcription-mediated amplification to wet mount microscopy, culture, and polymerase chain reaction for diagnosis of trichomoniasis in men and women. Am J Obstet Gynecol 2009;200:188.e1-7.

11. Loeffelholz MJ, Sanden GN. Bordetella. In: Murray PR, Baron EJ, Jorgensen JH, et al, editors. Manual of clinical microbiology. 9th edition. Washington, DC: ASM Press; 2007. p. 803–14.

12. Munson E, Napierala M, Munson KL, et al. Temporal characterization of carrot broth-enhanced real-time PCR as an alternative means for rapid detection of *Streptococcus agalactiae* from prenatal anorectal and vaginal screenings. J Clin Microbiol 2010;48:4495–500.

13. Ginocchio CC, Zhang F, Manji R, et al. Evaluation of multiple test methods for the detection of the novel 2009 influenza A (H1N1) during the New York City outbreak. J Clin Virol 2009;45:191–5.

14. Uyeki TM, Prasad R, Vukotich C, et al. Low sensitivity of rapid diagnostic test for influenza. Clin Infect Dis 2009;48:e89–92.

15. Mouton JW, Verkooyen R, van der Meijden WI, et al. Detection of *Chlamydia trachomatis* in male and female urine specimens by using the amplified *Chlamydia trachomatis* test. J Clin Microbiol 1997;35:1369–72.

16. Mahony J, Chong S, Jang D, et al. Urine specimens from pregnant and nonpregnant women inhibitory to amplification of *Chlamydia trachomatis* nucleic acid by PCR, ligase chain reaction, and transcription-mediated amplification: identification of urinary substances associated with inhibition and removal of inhibitory activity. J Clin Microbiol 1998;36:3122–6.

17. Verkooyen RP, Luijendijk A, Huisman WM, et al. Detection of PCR inhibitors in cervical specimens by using the AMPLICOR *Chlamydia trachomatis* assay. J Clin Microbiol 1996;34:3072–4.

18. Rosenstraus M, Wang Z, Chang SY, et al. An internal control for routine diagnostic PCR: design, properties, and effect on clinical performance. J Clin Microbiol 1998;36:191–7.

19. Monteiro L, Bonnemaison D, Vekris A, et al. Complex polysaccharides as PCR inhibitors in feces: *Helicobacter pylori* model. J Clin Microbiol 1997;35:995–8.

20. Schachter J, Moncada J, Liska S, et al. Nucleic acid amplification tests in the diagnosis of chlamydial and gonococcal infections of the oropharynx and rectum in men who have sex with men. Sex Transm Dis 2008;35:637–42.

21. Ota KV, Tamari IE, Smieja M, et al. Detection of *Neisseria gonorrhoeae* and *Chlamydia trachomatis* in pharyngeal and rectal specimens using the BD ProbeTec ET system, the Gen-Probe Aptima Combo 2 assay, and culture. Sex Transm Infect 2009;85:182–6.

22. Burd EM. Validation of laboratory-developed molecular assays for infectious diseases. Clin Microbiol Rev 2010;23:550–76.

23. Halling KC, Schrijver I, Persons DL. Test verification and validation for molecular diagnostic assays. Arch Pathol Lab Med 2012;136:11–3.

24. Centers for Disease Control and Prevention. 2015 Sexually transmitted diseases guidelines. Gonococcal infections. 2018. Available at: https://www.cdc.gov/std/tg2015/gonorrhea.htm. Accessed September 28, 2018.

25. Goodhart ME, Ogden J, Zaidi AA, et al. Factors affecting the performance of smear and culture tests for the detection of *Neisseria gonorrhoeae*. Sex Transm Dis 1982;9:63–9.

26. Atlas R, Snyder J. Reagents, stains, and media: bacteriology. In: Jorgensen JH, Pfaller MA, Carroll KC, et al, editors. Manual of clinical microbiology. 11th edition. Washington, DC: ASM Press; 2015. p. 316–49.

27. Martin JE Jr, Jackson RL. A biological environment chamber for the culture of *Neisseria gonorrhoeae*. J Am Vener Dis Assoc 1975;2:28–30.

28. Beverly A, Bailey-Griffin JR, Schwebke JR. InTray GC medium versus modified Thayer-Martin agar plates for diagnosis for gonorrhea from endocervical specimens. J Clin Microbiol 2000;38:3825–6.

29. Arbique JC, Forward KR, Leblanc J. Evaluation of four commercial transport media for the survival of *Neisseria gonorrhoeae*. Diagn Microbiol Infect Dis 2000;36:163–8.

30. Livengood CH III, Wrenn JW. Evaluation of COBAS AMPLICOR (Roche): accuracy in detection of *Chlamydia trachomatis* and *Neisseria gonorrhoeae* by coamplification of endocervical specimens. J Clin Microbiol 2001;39:2928–32.

31. Gaydos CA, Quinn TC, Willis D, et al. Performance of the APTIMA Combo 2 assay for detection of *Chlamydia trachomatis* and *Neisseria gonorrhoeae* in female urine and endocervical swab specimens. J Clin Microbiol 2003;41:304–9.

32. Lowe P, O'Loughlin P, Evans K, et al. Comparison of the Gen-Probe APTIMA Combo 2 assay to the AMPLICOR CT/NG assay for detection of *Chlamydia trachomatis* and *Neisseria gonorrhoeae* in urine samples from Australian men and women. J Clin Microbiol 2006;44:2619–21.

33. Centers for Disease Control and Prevention. 2015 Sexually transmitted diseases guidelines. Chlamydial infections. 2018. https://www.cdc.gov/std/tg2015/chlamydia.htm. Accessed September 28, 2018.

34. Chambers LC, Khosropour CM, Dombrowski JC, et al. Racial/ethnic disparities in the lifetime risk of *Chlamydia trachomatis* diagnosis and adverse reproductive health outcomes among women in King County, Washington. Clin Infect Dis 2018;67(4):593–9.

35. Smith TF. Comparative recoveries of *Chlamydia* from urethral specimens using glass vials and plastic microtiter plates. Am J Clin Pathol 1977;67:496–8.

36. Boyadzhyan B, Yashina T, Yatabe JH, et al. Comparison of the APTIMA CT and GC assays with the APTIMA Combo 2 assay, the Abbott LCx assay, and direct fluorescent-antibody and culture assays for detection of *Chlamydia trachomatis* and *Neisseria gonorrhoeae*. J Clin Microbiol 2004;42:3089–93.

37. Swain GR, McDonald RA, Pfister JR, et al. Decision analysis: point-of-care *Chlamydia* testing vs. laboratory-based methods. Clin Med Res 2004;2:29–35.

38. van der Pol B, Quinn TC, Gaydos CA, et al. Multicenter evaluation of the AMPLI-COR and automated COBAS AMPLICOR CT/NG tests for detection of *Chlamydia trachomatis*. J Clin Microbiol 2000;38:1105–12.

39. Farrell D. Evaluation of AMPLICOR *Neisseria gonorrhoeae* PCR using *cppB* nested PCR and 16S rRNA PCR. J Clin Microbiol 1999;37:386–90.

40. van der Pol B, Martin DH, Schachter J, et al. Enhancing the specificity of the CO-BAS AMPLICOR CT/NG test for *Neisseria gonorrhoeae* by retesting specimens with equivocal results. J Clin Microbiol 2001;39:3092–8.

41. Bachmann LH, Johnson RE, Cheng H, et al. Nucleic acid amplification tests for diagnosis of *Neisseria gonorrhoeae* oropharyngeal infections. J Clin Microbiol 2009;47:902–7.

42. Nagasawa Z, Ikeda-Dantsuji Y, Niwa T, et al. Evaluation of APTIMA Combo 2 for cross-reactivity with oropharyngeal *Neisseria* species and other microorganisms. Clin Chim Acta 2010;411:776–8.

43. Workowski KA, Bolan GA. Sexually transmitted diseases treatment guidelines, 2015. MMWR Recomm Rep 2015;64(3):20–1, 72-73.

44. Soni S, Horner P, Rayment M, et al. 2018 BASHH UK national guideline for the management of infection with *Mycoplasma genitalium*. 2017. Available at: https://www.bashhguidelines.org/media/1182/bashh-mgen-guideline-2018_draft-for-consultation.pdf. Accessed May 5, 2018.

45. Jensen JS, Cusini M, Gomberg M, et al. 2016 European guideline on *Mycoplasma genitalium* infections. J Eur Acad Dermatol Venereol 2016;(10):1650–6.

46. Lis R, Rowhani-Rahbar A, Manhart LE. *Mycoplasma genitalium* infection and female reproductive tract disease: a meta-analysis. Clin Infect Dis 2015;61:418–26.

47. Taylor-Robinson D, Jensen JS. *Mycoplasma genitalium*: from chrysalis to multicolored butterfly. Clin Microbiol Rev 2011;24:498–514.

48. Jensen JS, Hansen HT, Lind K. Isolation of *Mycoplasma genitalium* strains from the male urethra. J Clin Microbiol 1996;34:286–91.

49. Baseman JB, Cagle M, Korte JE, et al. Diagnostic assessment of *Mycoplasma genitalium* in culture-positive women. J Clin Microbiol 2004;42:203–11.

50. Taylor-Robinson D, Furr PM, Tully JG. Serological cross-reactions between *Mycoplasma genitalium* and *Mycoplasma pneumoniae*. Lancet 1983;1(8323):527.

51. Taylor-Robinson D, Furr PM, Hanna NF. Microbiological and serological study of non-gonococcal urethritis with special reference to *Mycoplasma genitalium*. Genitourin Med 1985;61:319–24.

52. Jacobs E, Watter T, Schaefer HE, et al. Comparison of host responses after intranasal infection of guinea pigs with *Mycoplasma genitalium* or *Mycoplasma pneumoniae*. Microb Pathog 1991;10:221–9.

53. Ma L, Mancuso M, Williams JA, et al. Extensive variation and rapid shift of the MG192 sequence in *Mycoplasma genitalium* strains from patients with chronic infection. Infect Immun 2014;82:1326–34.

54. Burgos R, Totten PA. MG428 is a novel positive regulator of recombination that triggers *mgpB* and *mgpC* gene variation in *Mycoplasma genitalium*. Mol Microbiol 2014;94:290–306.

55. Inamine JM, Loechel S, Collier AM, et al. Nucleotide sequence of the MgPa (mgp) operon of *Mycoplasma genitalium* and comparison to the P1 (mpp) operon of *Mycoplasma pneumoniae*. Gene 1989;82:259–67.

56. Munson E. Molecular diagnostics update for the emerging (if not already widespread) sexually-transmitted infection agent *Mycoplasma genitalium*: just about ready for prime time. J Clin Microbiol 2017;55:2894–902.

57. Napierala M, Munson E, Wenten D, et al. Detection of *Mycoplasma genitalium* from male primary urine specimens: an epidemiologic dichotomy with *Trichomonas vaginalis*. Diagn Microbiol Infect Dis 2015;82:194–8.
58. Munson E, Bykowski H, Munson KL, et al. Clinical laboratory assessment of *Mycoplasma genitalium* transcription-mediated amplification using primary female urogenital specimens. J Clin Microbiol 2016;54:432–8.
59. Chernesky M, Jang D, Smieja M, et al. Urinary meatal swabbing detects more men infected with *Mycoplasma genitalium* and four other sexually-transmitted infections than first catch urine. Sex Transm Dis 2017;44:489–91.
60. Tabrizi SN, Tan LY, Walker S, et al. Multiplex assay for simultaneous detection of *Mycoplasma genitalium* and macrolide resistance using Plexzyme and PlexPrime technology. PLoS One 2016;11:e0156740.
61. Getman D, Jiang A, O'Donnell M, et al. *Mycoplasma genitalium* prevalence, co-infection, and macrolide antibiotic resistance frequency in a multicenter clinical study cohort in the United States. J Clin Microbiol 2016;54:2278–83.
62. Schwebke JR. Trichomonas vaginalis. In: Mandell GL, Bennett JE, Dolin R, editors. Mandell, Douglas, and Bennett's principles and practice of infectious diseases. 7th edition. Philadelphia: Churchill Livingstone Elsevier, Inc; 2010. p. 3535–8.
63. Munson E, Napierala M, Munson KL. Update on laboratory diagnosis and epidemiology of *Trichomonas vaginalis*: you can teach an "old" dog "new" trichs. Clin Microbiol Newsl 2016;38:159–68.
64. Munson E, Napierala M, Olson R, et al. Impact of *Trichomonas vaginalis* transcription-mediated amplification-based analyte-specific-reagent testing in a metropolitan setting of high sexually transmitted disease prevalence. J Clin Microbiol 2008;46:3368–74.
65. McCann JS. Comparison of direct microscopy and culture in the diagnosis of trichomoniasis. Br J Vener Dis 1974;50:450–2.
66. Spence MR, Hollander DH, Smith J, et al. The clinical and laboratory diagnosis of *Trichomonas vaginalis* infection. Sex Transm Dis 1980;7:168–71.
67. Krieger JN, Tam MR, Stevens CE, et al. Diagnosis of trichomoniasis. Comparison of conventional wet-mount examination with cytologic studies, cultures, and monoclonal antibody staining of direct specimens. JAMA 1998;259:1223–7.
68. Garber GE, Sibau L, Ma R, et al. Cell culture compared with broth for detection of *Trichomonas vaginalis*. J Clin Microbiol 1987;25:1275–9.
69. Fouts AC, Kraus SJ. *Trichomonas vaginalis*: reevaluation of its clinical presentation and laboratory diagnosis. J Infect Dis 1980;141:137–43.
70. Levi MH, Torres J, Piña C, et al. Comparison of the InPouch TV culture system and Diamond's modified medium for detection of *Trichomonas vaginalis*. J Clin Microbiol 1997;35:3308–10.
71. Huppert JS, Mortensen JE, Reed JL, et al. Rapid antigen testing compares favorably with transcription-mediated amplification assay for the detection of *Trichomonas vaginalis* in young women. Clin Infect Dis 2007;45:194–8.
72. Munson KL, Napierala M, Munson E. Suboptimal *Trichomonas vaginalis* antigen test performance in a low-prevalence sexually transmitted infection community. J Clin Microbiol 2016;54:500–1.
73. Andrea SB, Chapin KC. Comparison of Aptima *Trichomonas vaginalis* transcription-mediated amplification assay and BD Affirm VPIII for detection of *Trichomonas vaginalis* in symptomatic women: performance parameters and epidemiological implications. J Clin Microbiol 2011;49:866–9.

74. Cartwright CP, Lembke BD, Ramachandran K, et al. Comparison of nucleic acid amplification assays with BD Affirm VPIII for diagnosis of vaginitis in symptomatic women. J Clin Microbiol 2013;51:3694–9.

75. Munson E, Napierala M, Schell RF. Insights into trichomoniasis as a result of highly sensitive molecular diagnostics screening in a high-prevalence sexually transmitted infection community. Expert Rev Anti Infect Ther 2013;11:845–63.

76. Kirby T. *Mycoplasma genitalium*: a potential new superbug. Lancet 2018;18(9): 951–2.

Cardiac Laboratory Markers

Joshua L. Waynick, MMS, PA-C

KEYWORDS

- Cardiac markers • Troponin • BNP • NT-proBNP

KEY POINTS

- Troponin is the gold standard for evaluation of cardiac myocyte damage.
- Interpretation of troponin continues to evolve with a new definition of myocardial injury.
- B-type natriuretic peptide (BNP) and BNP molecule and the N-terminal component BNP are most helpful in evaluation of dyspnea but can also serve a role in evaluating acute on chronic heart failure.

The main components of laboratory testing in cardiology consist of serum markers for cardiac myocyte damage and volume overload. Despite their widespread use, these markers should only aid in clarifying the clinical picture and should not be used to exclusively make a diagnosis. Myocyte damage is evaluated with troponin, and there are nuances to troponin interpretation. Considerations include the timing of symptom onset, when the sample is drawn, and the differential diagnosis for elevated cardiac troponin. Volume overload is evaluated with natriuretic peptide markers. These markers are most commonly ordered for evaluation of possible heart failure, but may be useful in other conditions as well. Considerations for natriuretic peptide markers include understanding the difference between normal values and cutoffs for the diagnosis of heart failure as well as the differential diagnosis for an elevated level.

MARKERS FOR CARDIAC MYOCYTE DAMAGE

Cardiac biomarkers in the bloodstream are released from cardiac myocytes due to necrosis and cell death. Medical conditions that only cause transient ischemia without any necrosis would not cause biomarker elevation. Early tests for damage included creatine kinase, creatine kinase muscle/brain, myoglobin, and cardiac troponin. All of these markers, except cardiac troponin, are nonspecific for cardiac cells and can be found in multiple tissue types throughout the body, making them less preferred than cardiac troponin. Troponin I and T are more specific for cardiac myocyte necrosis

Disclosure Statement: No disclosures.
Department of PA Studies, Wake Forest School of Medicine, Medical Center Boulevard, Winston Salem, NC 27157, USA
E-mail address: jwaynick@wakehealth.edu

and are currently the gold standard for evaluating damage. The tests used to evaluate for cardiac damage continue to evolve, as do the criteria for interpreting them and the nomenclature used to interpret and discuss the results.

TROPONIN ANATOMY AND PHYSIOLOGY

The troponin molecule is a protein that is found in skeletal and cardiac muscle but is absent in smooth muscle. There are 3 forms of troponin: I, C, and T. These molecules are bound to tropomyosin and in their resting state block the attachment of myosin to its binding site on actin. When troponin is activated by calcium, it undergoes a configuration change allowing myosin to bind to actin. Most of cardiac troponin is found bound within these protein complexes, but some is found unbound within the cell. During cardiac cell necrosis, troponin that is free in the cytoplasm will leak out of the cells first, causing an initial early increase. This increase is then followed by ongoing leak from the destruction of bound proteins within the cell. The cardiac form of troponin I is found only in heart muscle, whereas troponin T is found in both cardiac muscle and some skeletal muscle.

TROPONIN ASSAYS

Cardiac troponin I or T samples are obtained via venous blood samples, which then undergo immunoassay testing by point-of-care or formal laboratory testing. Immunoassay testing uses monoclonal antibodies that bind to a specific target. The bound antibodies can then be measured and quantified. The use of monoclonal antibodies leads to variability in testing because each monoclonal antibody binds to a specific site in the amino acid sequence. Troponin molecules circulate in degraded forms as they are released during cell death. If the specific amino acid sequence that a particular monoclonal antibody binds to is disrupted by the degradation of the molecule, then the monoclonal antibody is unable to bind, and some troponin will not be detected.[1] Degradation of troponin leads to variability of results between assays.

Understanding when a single cardiac troponin level can be used as opposed to serial measurements is a key distinction. Troponins can be repeated within 3 to 6 hours of the first draw when using contemporary assays, or sooner if using a high-sensitivity assay. Noting the timing of chest pain onset is also important. For example, if a patient comes in with several hours of typical angina and a single positive troponin, a trend is less necessary for diagnosis because the elevated troponin indicates cardiac myocyte damage has occurred. However, the trend may help with prognosis, because higher levels of troponins are associated with a greater degree of damage and therefore a worse prognosis. The trend would be essential in a patient who experiences typical angina for only minutes before the level is drawn. Incorrectly interpreting a troponin level drawn within minutes of chest pain onset may lead to incorrect diagnosis, improper treatment, and ultimately, a poor outcome for the patient. The trend is also important when a troponin is ordered for symptoms other than angina or angina equivalents, or when the suspicion for myocardial infarction is low. An elevated troponin in this scenario could be due to a variety of reasons, and the trend could be helpful in narrowing the differential.

Currently, there is no clear standardization of troponin I or T assays, mainly due to the lack of a control or reference sample.[1] Cardiac troponin testing is standardized through the ability to measure a level that is greater than the 99th percentile upper reference limit (URL) of a healthy population. How the 99th percentile URL is decided and who makes up the healthy population used to develop the URL lack standardization, so it varies between manufacturers.[2] Notably, the 99th percentile URL method does not take into account variation in levels, which may occur with normal aging.[1] There has been work to increase quality of measurements as well as to guide the creation of a reference material; however, this work is ongoing.[1] In order to improve troponin assay standardization, efforts need to be made to ensure that the healthy population used to create the 99th percentile URL is truly healthy. Multiple methods have been used or proposed for verifying that a subject is "healthy" before using them in a study to create the 99th percentile URL for an assay.[3] Some possibilities include additional laboratory work or cardiac imaging, but these are not always used in studies due to cost concerns.[3] Given the variability in cardiac troponin assays, values from different assays should not be joined together to create a trend.[2] Without having a clear method for determining the 99th percentile URL, an overestimation or underestimation of normal levels of cardiac troponin may continue to occur with ongoing high levels of variability between assays.

There are 3 types of cardiac troponin testing: point of care, contemporary, and high sensitivity. Contemporary and high-sensitivity assays are quantitative, whereas point-of-care tests may be either qualitative or quantitative. Understanding which style of cardiac troponin testing is used by a clinical laboratory is important due to wide variation in sensitivity. Point-of-care and contemporary assays are less likely to be able to pick up variations within the 99th percentile.[2] Also, these assays are less likely to detect levels that are just over the threshold of positive.[2] The newer high-sensitivity cardiac troponin assays were developed to address some of these limitations. The current definition of high-sensitivity cardiac troponin assays is that these tests should have a detectable level of troponin in greater than 50% of the patients below the 99th percentile.[4] The term "high sensitivity" does not deal with clinical sensitivity but instead with analytical sensitivity. Analytical sensitivity refers to how well the test detects troponin in a sample, even at lower concentrations. The clinical sensitivity for acute myocardial infarction relies on proper ordering practices and avoiding overordering cardiac troponin levels without the appropriate clinical context.

DIFFERENTIAL DIAGNOSIS FOR ELEVATED TROPONIN

As cardiac troponin becomes more sensitive to any type of myocardial damage, consideration of the full differential diagnosis for elevated levels is important, especially when the test is being ordered without the typical symptoms of ischemic myocardial damage. **Table 1** gives a complete list of the differential for elevated cardiac troponin levels, which is typically split into 3 main groups: ischemic, nonischemic, and analytical. The differential can broadly be split into plaque instability or rupture, supply versus demand mismatch, structural heart disease/damage, and systemic disease processes. In the absence of any of these causes of cardiac troponin elevation, an analytical issue should be considered and discussed with the resulting laboratory.

DEFINITION OF ACUTE MYOCARDIAL INJURY/INFARCTION WITH FOCUS ON TROPONIN

The fourth universal definition of myocardial infarction delineates myocardial injury from myocardial infarction using cardiac troponin as well as clinical signs and symptoms of ischemia.[2] Any elevation of cardiac troponin without evidence of ischemia is considered a myocardial injury. Myocardial injury can be diagnosed when cardiac troponin increases to above the 99th percentile URL cutoff, and then the trend can be used to determine if the elevation is due to acute injury or chronic disease.[2] An elevated cardiac troponin level, which remains unchanged on serial measurements, would be representative of chronic disease as opposed to a level that trends upwards

Table 1		
Differential diagnosis for elevated troponin		
Ischemic	**Nonischemic**	**Analytical**
ACS	Cardiac	Poor assay performance
STEMI	Heart failure	Calibration error
Non-STEMI	Viral cardiomyopathy	Heterophile antibodies
Not ACS	Pericarditis/myocarditis	Interfering substance
Coronary cause	Electrical shock	
Increased demand	Surgery	
Hypertension	Radiofrequency ablation	
Spasm	Malignancy	
Embolism	Stress cardiomyopathy	
Procedure related	Infiltrative disease	
Percutaneous intervention	Systemic disease	
Cardiac surgery	Pulmonary embolus	
Cocaine/methamphetamine	Anthracycline toxicity	
Noncoronary cause	Blunt trauma	
Hypoxia	Volume overload	
Global ischemia	Renal failure	
Hypoperfusion	Sepsis	
Cardiac surgery	Stroke	
	Subarachnoid hemorrhage	

Adapted from Newby LK, Jesse RL, Babb JD, et al. ACCF 2012 expert consensus document on practical clinical considerations in the interpretation of troponin elevations. J Am Coll Cardiol 2012;60:2427–63.

and is suggestive of an acute process. Myocardial infarction is identified when cardiac troponin levels increase above the 99th percentile URL, and there are correlating clinical signs or symptoms of myocardial ischemia.[2] If myocardial ischemia is occurring, then the appropriate type of myocardial infarction should be diagnosed using the electrocardiogram.

EVALUATION OF TROPONIN LEVEL WITH CLINICAL AND DIAGNOSTIC CORRELATION

Cardiac troponin is a single tool in diagnosing acute myocardial infarction and should always be reviewed within the context of the patient's case to ensure appropriate utilization. Cardiac troponin assays are becoming more analytically sensitive but lack standardization of the 99th percentile URL. Because the fourth universal definition of myocardial infarction defines the difference between myocardial injury versus myocardial infarction, providers should also think in these terms. Thorough review of the differential diagnoses for chest pain and consideration of the patient's pretest probability for ischemia and infarction based on history are key to appropriate ordering and interpretation. When cardiac troponin is elevated but without a clear cause, the differential for ordering should be reviewed. A cardiac troponin level should also be interpreted in context of other diagnostics, such as electrocardiography and echocardiography as well as radionuclide imaging, cardiac magnetic resonance, or coronary angiography.

NOVEL CARDIAC MARKERS

There is continued research into alternative markers for cardiac damage beyond cardiac troponins. Some currently discussed markers for direct cardiac myocyte damage include ischemia-modified albumin (IMA) and heart-type fatty acid binding protein (hFABP). During ischemic episodes, the N-terminal portion of albumin is modified by the products of ischemia, which can then be detected through a binding assay. IMA is unique because it is created through ischemia as opposed to necrosis, making it a potential marker for angina, and IMA can be detected soon after an ischemic episode.[5] However, IMA is nonspecific due to the fact that anything that causes ischemia will create IMA.

Another unique marker for cardiac damage is hFABP, which is found primarily in cardiac myocytes as a component of fatty acid metabolism and is released rapidly after damage to the cell.[6] hFABP is primarily found in cardiac myocytes so it is more specific for cardiac myocyte necrosis. One recent trial compared the utility of IMA and hFABP versus cardiac troponin for myocardial infarction after coronary artery bypass grafting.[6] This trial showed that hFABP was more sensitive than IMA for detecting postoperative myocardial infarction and was detected sooner than cardiac troponin I.[6] However, another large trial showed that hFABP did not aid in the diagnosis of non-ST elevated myocardial infarctions over cardiac troponin.[7] Although cardiac troponin remains the gold standard in diagnosis of cardiac myocyte damage, these new markers may serve useful in angina or be used in a multimodal approach to improve the sensitivity of troponin early in acute myocardial infarction. However, it is unlikely that cardiac troponin will be supplanted as the marker of choice.[5]

MARKER FOR VOLUME OVERLOAD

The other way that laboratory medicine is used in the evaluation of cardiac patients is through markers of volume overload. The brain natriuretic peptide or B-type natriuretic peptide (BNP) can be used to help build the case for the diagnosis of heart failure within the appropriate clinical scenarios. The heart produces 2 types of natriuretic peptides: atria natriuretic peptide (ANP) and BNP. The clinical importance of ANP is less clear, and a test has only recently become available to measure ANP.[1] BNP has clear clinical utility. This section reviews BNP's anatomy and physiology, the process of obtaining a BNP, differential diagnosis for elevated concentrations, clinical use, and variations in interpretation.

ANATOMY AND PHYSIOLOGY OF B-TYPE NATRIURETIC PEPTIDE

Ventricular myocyte cells produce a pro-BNP molecule that is activated before secretion. The pro-BNP molecule is separated into 2 parts, the physiologically active BNP molecule and the N-terminal component (NT-proBNP), which is not physiologically active. In a state of normal health, BNP secretion occurs due to an increase in ventricular stretch from increased volume. Once BNP is secreted by the ventricle, it rapidly acts to increase sodium excretion from the kidneys, a process known as natriuresis, as well as to decrease systemic vascular resistance. In heart failure, the myocytes inappropriately secrete large amounts of pro-BNP, the precursor to BNP, in addition to smaller amounts of BNP and NT-proBNP. Pro-BNP does not affect natriuresis or systematic vascular resistance, contributing to volume overload.

HOW MARKERS ARE OBTAINED AND INTERPRETED

NT-proBNP is measured from plasma, whereas BNP is measured from whole blood. Quantification of the BNP or NT-proBNP level occurs using immunoassays that target specific portions of each molecule. The precursor molecule pro-BNP contains the specific areas targeted by antibodies for either the BNP or the NT-proBNP assay, and therefore, any pro-BNP that is found in the bloodstream will be detected and quantified by either assay type.[1]

The cutoff for either BNP or NT-proBNP assays continues to be studied and refined because both can be affected by gender, ethnicity, age, and cardiac disease other than heart failure.[1] Currently, the normal value for BNP assays is less than 100 pg/mL for all ages. The cutoff for NT-proBNP is set at less than 125 pg/mL for patients less than 75 years and less than 450 pg/mL for patients greater than 75 years.[1] However, the normal values and the values where heart failure is accurately diagnosed are different, causing gray areas. The BNP cutoff where heart failure can be ruled in as a diagnosis is 400 pg/mL; therefore, dyspnea in patient with a BNP less than 400 pg/mL is less likely to be from heart failure. NT-proBNP also has cutoffs for the diagnosis of heart failure, which varies from its normal. Age differences are also reflected in the level whereby heart failure can be diagnosed: less than 50 years old (450 pg/mL), 50 to 75 years old (900 pg/mL), and greater than 75 years old (1800 pg/mL).[8] An NT-proBNP of less than 300 pg/nL has a strong negative predictive value for heart failure.[8]

DIFFERENTIAL DIAGNOSIS AND CLINICAL CONTEXT

When ordered in the appropriate clinical context, an elevated BNP or NT-proBNP can help suggest the diagnosis of heart failure with reduced ejection fraction or heart failure with preserved ejection fraction, either of which could be acute or chronic. Disease states other than heart failure (see Table 2 in Ref.[9]) can cause elevation in BNP. Given this differential, careful consideration to the underlying cause of a patient's elevated BNP or NT-proBNP is necessary before attributing the elevation to heart failure.

CLINICAL CONTEXT

The common clinical scenario for ordering a BNP or NT-proBNP level is for further evaluation of a patient with dyspnea who has an unclear cause in either the ambulatory or emergency department settings.[10] A normal BNP or NT-proBNP concentration has a high negative predictive value, helping to exclude the diagnosis of heart failure. The positive predictive value of an elevated BNP or NT-proBNP level is not as helpful given the variety of conditions that can cause elevation, but does improve if the value is above the cutoff point where heart failure can be ruled in. Patients who are at risk for developing either type of heart failure may benefit from BNP or NT-proBNP screening.[10] An elevated level, regardless of symptoms, could prompt additional testing, such as cardiac imaging, to identify patients at the earliest stages of heart failure, allowing for prompt initiation of treatment.[10] There is no clear standard at this time for how frequently these markers should be monitored in a patient who is at risk for heart failure.

Another clinical scenario being researched is tracking the treatment of heart failure using serial BNP or NT-proBNP levels. The thought process is that if BNP is secreted due to increased ventricular pressure and volume overload, then as the volume overload state improves, the natriuretic peptide concentrations should trend down toward baseline. However, the current heart failure guidelines do not recommend this approach.[10] A recent meta-analysis determined that the overall quality of the evidence for natriuretic peptide–guided therapy is low and showed unclear benefit on mortality and patient's quality of life.[9] It did however show a possible improvement in the rate of readmission for decompensation.[9]

Although the clinical utility of tracking natriuretic peptides to monitor the efficacy of treatment is unclear, there is utility in using natriuretic peptides to provide prognosis in heart failure. Using BNP to aid in prognosis is supported by the current heart failure guidelines as well as the 2017 update.[10] Checking a natriuretic peptide on initial presentation to the hospital with an acute decompensation will give an idea of the disease severity and provide an estimation of mortality during the hospitalization as higher levels portend a higher risk of mortality.[10] Another area that may be useful would be checking a level at the time of discharge. This allows for the trend during hospitalization to be evaluated, possibly giving information regarding the effectiveness of treatment as well as post-discharge prognosis, including risk of readmission.[10] This recommendation is not for medication-guided natriuretic peptide therapy, or aiming for a certain peptide level, only assisting in the discussion regarding prognosis.[10]

Natriuretic peptides may also serve to provide prognosis and risk stratification for patients beyond those with heart failure, including those with an acute coronary syndrome (ACS) as well as hypertrophic cardiomyopathy (HCM). One recent study in patients with type 2 diabetes mellitus and an ACS process showed that a baseline BNP or an NT-proBNP level can be used to estimate the risk of heart failure, additional myocardial infarctions, stroke, and death.[11] Another recent trial analyzed NT-proBNP data from the time of admission for acute myocardial infarction and from 1 month after the event.[12] Analysis showed that patients with persistently elevated levels 1 month after the event were at a higher risk of mortality.[12] In a study evaluating patients with HCM, it was found that a higher BNP level correlates with an increase in symptoms as well as an increased likelihood of requiring invasive intervention.[13] Given that BNP levels reflect possible physiologic compromise, it may also serve to help risk-stratify patients who have sepsis. One meta-analysis has shown that elevated BNP levels in patients with sepsis increases risk of mortality.[14]

PATIENT FACTORS THAT COMPLICATE NATRIURETIC PEPTIDE INTERPRETATION

Common factors that may affect the interpretation of BNP levels include obesity, age, and renal disease. Typically, as the body mass index trends into the obese range, the levels of BNP will start to decrease.[15] Several mechanisms have been proposed for this relationship, including kidney hyperfiltration, increased clearance by adipocytes, and hyperinsulinemia directly affecting BNP secretion.[15] NT-proBNP can be applied with the same cutoffs for possible heart failure, whereas BNP should be applied using a lower normal.[15] As mentioned earlier, age must be considered when using NT-proBNP levels, in that levels tend to increase with age. Renal failure will lead to an accumulation of BNP and NT-proBNP irrespective of heart failure and therefore is less helpful in these patients. However, the negative predictive value of BNP still holds if the value is normal for these patients. A final consideration is that natriuretic peptide concentrations in general are higher in women than in men. BNP and NT-proBNP are useful markers in the diagnosis of heart failure, but caution should be used in certain patients.

SUMMARY

The general availability of troponin and natriuretic peptides makes them easy to order in the setting of a suspected cardiac disorder. However, these tests have several considerations that should be reviewed when interpreting results. Troponin interpretation hinges on the timing of symptom onset, when the sample was drawn, and the differences between myocardial injury and myocardial infarction. There is an extensive list of possible diagnoses for an elevated troponin. If a myocardial infarction is not occurring, then evaluation for other disease processes is necessary. Interpretation of BNP or NT-proBNP is more complex and relies on knowledge of normal values, which for

NT-proBNP varies by age as well as the heart-failure diagnosis cut points. If an NT-proBNP is elevated above normal but is below the designated heart failure cutoffs, a diagnosis of heart failure should not be made and the differential should be revisited. Misapplication of these markers leads to errors, such as misdiagnosing, initiation of potentially dangerous medications, and premature discharge. Appropriate ordering after evaluating pretest probability is the best way to improve clinical sensitivity.

REFERENCES

1. Apple FS, Goetze JP, Jaffe AS. Cardiac function. In: Nader R, editor. Tietz textbook of clinical chemistry and molecular diagnostics. 6th edition. St Louis (MO): Elsevier; 2018. p. 1201–55.e17.
2. Thygesen K, Alpert JS, Jaffe AS, et al. Fourth universal definition of myocardial infarction. J Am Coll Cardiol 2018;72:2231–64.
3. Sandoval Y, Apple FS. The global need to define normality: the 99th percentile value of cardiac troponin. Clin Chem 2014;60:455–62.
4. Sherwood MW, Newby K. High-sensitivity troponin assays: evidence, indications, and reasonable use. J Am Heart Assoc 2014;3. https://doi.org/10.1161/JAHA.113.000403.
5. Spencer TR, Sidhu MS, Bisaillon J, et al. Novel cardiac biomarkers for emergency department evaluation of acute coronary syndrome: the recent evidence on non-troponin biomarkers and their limitations. Curr Emerg Hosp Med Rep 2016;4:99–106.
6. Thielmann M, Pasa S, Holst T, et al. Heart-type fatty acid binding protein and ischemia-modified albumin for detection of myocardial infarction after coronary artery bypass graft surgery. Ann Thorac Surg 2017;104:130–7.
7. Reiter M, Twerenbold R, Reichlin T, et al. Heart-type fatty acid-binding protein in the early diagnosis of acute myocardial infarction. Heart 2013;99:708–14.
8. Januzzi JL, Chen-Tournoux AA, Christenson RH, et al. N-terminal pro-B-type natriuretic peptide in the emergency department: the ICON-RELOADED study. J Am Coll Cardiol 2018;71:1191–200.
9. Yancy CW, Jessup M, Bozkurt B, et al. 2017 ACC/AHA/HFSA focused update of the 2013 ACCF/AHA guideline for the management of heart failure. Circulation 2017;136:e137–61.
10. McLellan J, Heneghan CJ, Perera R, et al. B-type natriuretic peptide-guided treatment for heart failure. Cochrane Database Syst Rev 2016;(12):CD008966.
11. Wolsk E, Claggett B, Pfeffer M, et al. Role of B-type natriuretic peptide and N-terminal prohormone BNP as predictors of cardiovascular morbidity and mortality in patients with a recent coronary event and type 2 diabetes mellitus. J Am Heart Assoc 2017;6. https://doi.org/10.1161/JAHA.116.004743.
12. Kontos MC, Lanfear DE, Gosch K, et al. Prognostic value of serial N-terminal pro-brain natriuretic peptide testing in patients with acute myocardial infarction. Am J Cardiol 2017;120:181–5.
13. Geske JB, McKie PM, Ommen SR, et al. B-type natriuretic peptide and survival in hypertrophic cardiomyopathy. J Am Coll Cardiol 2013;61:2456–60.
14. Wang F, Wu Y, Tang L, et al. Brain natriuretic peptide for prediction of mortality in patients with sepsis: a systematic review and meta-analysis. Crit Care 2012;16:R74.
15. Madamanchi C, Alhosani H, Sumida A, et al. Obesity and natriuretic peptides, BNP and NT-proBNP: mechanisms and diagnostics implications for heart failure. Int J Cardiol 2014;176:611–7.

Thyroid Testing and Interpretation

Molly Paulson, DHSc, MPAS, PA-C, MT (ASCP)

KEYWORDS

- Thyroid disease • Thyroid hormones • Thyroid testing
- Hypothalmic-pituitary-thyroid (HPT) axis

KEY POINTS

- Thyrotropin (TSH) is the initial test of choice for assessing thyroid function, followed by free thyroxine (fT4) in the setting of an otherwise normally functioning HPT axis.
- If thyroiditis is suspected, antibody testing is warranted.
- If TSH, fT4, and antibody testing do not fully explain the patient presentation, clinicians should investigate anomalies in the thyroid binding globulin carrier proteins and thyroid resistance to normal hormonal stimulation.
- Exploration of other neuroendocrine pathologic conditions or anomalies within the hypothalamus or pituitary gland should be considered if the thyroid gland appears anatomically and physiologically intact.

INTRODUCTION

The thyroid gland produces, stores, and secretes 3 active hormones: thyroxine (T4), triiodothyronine (T3), and calcitonin (**Table 1**). It also produces thyroglobulin (TG), a tyrosine-rich glycoprotein (**Table 2**). TG, along with iodine, is essential to synthesize T3 and T4, known collectively as thyroid hormone. Thyroid hormone and TG are produced in the follicular cells of the thyroid gland. Calcitonin, the third thyroid hormone, is produced in the parafollicular cells and functions to maintain calcium homeostasis by decreasing osteoclast activity in the bone and by increasing urinary excretion of calcium. Calcitonin is often used to monitor progression and treatment of thyroid cancer.[1–3] Thyroid hormones, primarily T3, control metabolic activity within individual cells throughout the body.[4,5]

Production and secretion of thyroid hormone are controlled by hormonal feedback between the hypothalamus, pituitary, and thyroid (HPT) glands (**Fig. 1**). Homeostasis

Disclosure statement: The author has no commercial or financial conflicts of interest or any funding sources to disclose.
College of Health Professions, 218 Cook-DeVos Center for Health Sciences, 301 Michigan St NE, Grand Rapids, MI 49503-3314, USA
E-mail address: paulsonm@gvsu.edu

Physician Assist Clin 4 (2019) 527–539
https://doi.org/10.1016/j.cpha.2019.02.006
2405-7991/19/© 2019 Elsevier Inc. All rights reserved.

Table 1
Hormones and hormone testing

Hormone	Laboratory Test	Description Details
Calcitonin	Calcitonin	• Inhibits bone resorption and increases urinary excretion of calcium • Increased in medullary thyroid cancer, neuroendocrine tumors, thyroiditis, pregnancy, newborns, and with some medications • Used to monitor progression or treatment of thyroid cancer, or noncancerous C-cell hyperplasia
T3	Total T3	• Total T3 includes bound and unbound T3 • Affected by circulating levels of thyroid binding globulin (TBG)
	fT3	• fT3 measures unbound levels of T3 • Results unaffected by thyroid-binding protein levels
TSH	TSH	• Most commonly ordered and most sensitive test of thyroid function • Ordered to diagnose thyroid malfunction, monitor thyroid replacement therapy, and monitor antithyroid treatment • Acute illness may affect results; testing should be avoided in ill or hospitalized patients
TRH	TRH stimulating test	• Inhibited by T4, T3, somatotropin, dopamine, and other hormones/medications • TRH stimulating test: Used to evaluate for hyperthyroidism when the TSH level is equivocal ○ An increase in the level of TSH following administration of TRH excludes secondary hypothyroidism or hyperthyroidism
T4	Total T4	• T4 converts to the more metabolically active T3 intracellularly • Results affected by circulating levels of TBG
	fT4	• Ordered if abnormal TSH to help detect, diagnose, and distinguish types of thyroid disease, monitor treatment efficacy, or TSH-sensitive thyroid cancers • Results affected by pregnancy, estrogen, medications, liver disease, systemic illness, pituitary dysfunction

Data from Refs.[1–3,8,10,12,18]

within the HPT axis optimizes cellular function throughout the body. Anatomic or physiologic abnormalities within the HPT axis can lead to significant morbidity.

Thyroid disease is the most common cause of HPT disruption and is frequently encountered.[6] According to the American Thyroid Association, "more than 12% of the US population will develop thyroid disease during their lifetime." Up to 60% will go undiagnosed.[7] Thyroid disease symptoms are nonspecific and are often seen in other disease processes.[8] Symptoms may include fatigue, skin changes, temperature intolerance, weight changes, cardiac dysrhythmias, gastrointestinal disturbances, weakness, myalgias, and slowed cognition. Thyroid dysfunction, in severe cases, can lead to death.[9,10] Clinicians need to be able to order and interpret the appropriate tests when thyroid disease is suspected.

After a review of the HPT axis, common thyroid diseases are discussed, including expected test results. Case histories highlight the complexity of thyroid disease and lead to a discussion of laboratory testing and interpretation. Tables provide a quick reference on each topic.

Table 2
Antibodies, carrier proteins, and catalysts

Antibodies, Proteins	Tests	Description Details
TG	TG	• A major autoantigen for autoimmune thyroiditis • Ordered to monitor thyroid disease treatment and progression, to help differentiate subacute thyroiditis and thyrotoxicosis factitia • Results affected by dietary supplements, especially biotin: avoid biotin for 12 h before blood draw • Test results negated by the presence of TGAb in the blood
TPOAb	TPOAb	• Found in both GD and Hashimoto thyroiditis
TGAb	TGAb	• Ordered to determine if TG can be used for monitoring progression/treatment of thyroid cancer ○ If TGAb are present, TG cannot be used

TSH receptor antibodies	TSHRAb
	○ Thyroid stimulating immunoglobulin (TSI)
	○ Thyroid binding inhibitory immunoglobulin (TBII)
		• Attach to TSH receptors in the thyroid gland
		  ○ TSI stimulates production of thyroid hormone leading to GD
		  ○ TBII blocks TSH from binding to receptors on the follicular cells leading to hypothyroidism

TPO		• A major autoantigen for autoimmune thyroiditis
TBG	TBG	• Produced by the liver • Transports thyroid hormone in bloodstream

Abbreviation: TSHRAb, TSH receptor antibodies.
Data from Refs.[1–3,10,14,16]

THE HYPOTHALAMUS, PITUITARY, AND THYROID AXIS

The hypothalamus is located ventrally in the forebrain. It produces thyrotropin releasing hormone (TRH) when thyroid levels are low, which stimulates the pituitary to release thyrotropin which is also known as thyroid stimulating hormone (TSH). TRH is regulated primarily by thyroid hormone, but also by somatostatin and dopamine (see **Table 1**).[11,12]

The pituitary gland is connected to the hypothalamus by the pituitary stalk. The anterior pituitary produces, stores, and releases several hormones, including TSH. The pituitary stalk provides both humoral and neural feedback between the 2 glands.[13]

The thyroid is located ventral to the trachea overlying the second to fourth tracheal rings. It is composed of 2 lobes, an isthmus, and occasionally, a pyramidal lobe. Underneath the thyroid gland are 4 parathyroid glands and the recurrent laryngeal nerves. These structures are important considerations when surgery in this area is being considered (**Table 3**).

THYROID FOLLICLES

Thyroid follicles (**Fig. 2**) are the primary functional units of the thyroid gland and produce both thyroid hormone and TG. The follicle is made up of thyrocytes packed tightly around a central lumen (see **Fig. 2**). This lumen serves as a reservoir for a colloidal mixture of TG, tyrosine fractions, thyroid hormone precursors, and T3 and T4.[14]

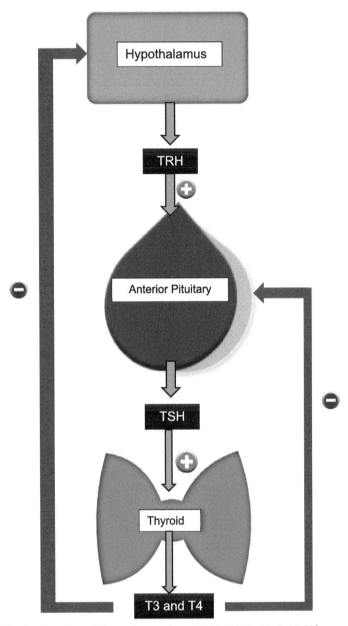

Fig. 1. HPT axis. (*Courtesy of* Susan Raaymakers, DHSc, MPAS, PA-C, RDCS.)

Iodine, an essential component of thyroid hormone, is transported to and catalyzed by membrane-bound thyroid peroxidase (TPO) into iodide and bound to TG or to tyrosyl residues (see **Table 2**). Iodinated tyrosyl residues are then converted into either monoiodothyronine or diiodothyronine and coupled to become either T3 or T4. Thyroid hormone is then stored within the lumen until needed.[15]

When needed, thyroid hormone is actively transported from the lumen, through the follicle (**Fig. 3**), and absorbed into the adjacent capillaries. High thyroid

Table 3
Pathologic processes (alphabetical)

Pathologic Process	Expected Test Results	Description Details
Apathetic hyperthyroidism	↓TSH, ↑fT4	• In elderly, multiple comorbidities blunt signs and symptoms of thyroid hormone excess
Euthyroid sick syndrome	↑TSH, ↓fT4	• Low thyroid levels in ill patients with a normal HPT axis • Thyroid testing and replacement typically not indicated
GD, diffuse thyroid hyperplasia	↓TSH & ↑fT4 ↑fT3 > ↑fT4 ↑TSHRAb	• TSH-like antibodies stimulate excessive production and secretion of thyroid hormone • RAIU: Increased uptake in a diffuse pattern (see **Table 4**)
Hashimoto thyroiditis, autoimmune thyroiditis	↑TSH, ↓fT4 ↑ Autoantibodies	• TPOAb (95% of cases), TGAb, TSHRAb • Lymphocytes infiltrate and destroy the thyroid follicles • Release of stored T3 and T4 followed by decreased production
Hyperthyroidism	↓TSH & ↑fT4	• Based on clinical symptoms, low TSH, and elevated fT4 • Secondary hyperthyroidism is thyrotoxicosis arising from a nonthyroid source
Hypothyroidism	↑TSH, ↓fT4	• Decreased production of thyroid hormone by the thyroid gland due to a variety of pathologic conditions • Based on clinical symptoms, elevated TSH level, and low fT4
Iatrogenic hypothyroidism	↑TSH, ↓fT4	• Hypofunctioning of the thyroid follicles caused by chemical, radiologic, or mechanical damage or interference. It may be intentional or unintentional
Myxedema crisis[12]	↑TSH, ↓fT4 ↓fT3	• Severe decompensated hypothyroidism characterized low cellular levels of T3
Postpartum thyroiditis	Initially: ↓TSH & ↑fT4 Subsequently: ↑TSH, ↓fT4 ↑TPOAb (usually) ↓RAIU	• Self-limited with a nontender goiter • Initial symptoms of hyperthyroidism (due to follicular disruption) followed by transient hypothyroidism • No follicular destruction
Subacute hypothyroidism	↑TSH normal fT4 ± autoantibodies	• Controversial diagnosis • Autoantibodies may or may not be present
Subacute thyroiditis	Initially: ↓TSH & ↑fT4 Subsequently: ↑TSH, ↓fT4 ↓RAIU	• Acute, inflammatory, self-limited (months) thyroiditis • Initial symptoms of hyperthyroidism (due to follicular disruption) followed by transient hypothyroidism • Diagnosis confirmed with decreased RAIU • Thyroid-associated antibodies are usually negative

(continued on next page)

Pathologic Process	Expected Test Results	Description Details
Table 3 *(continued)*		
Thyroid cancers	Thyroid hormone tests variable U/S, FNA, RAIU	• Several types • Requires imaging and biopsy for confirmation
Thyroiditis	↓TSH & ↑fT4	• Acute or chronic, painful or painless, inflammation of the thyroid gland • May be idiopathic or caused by autoimmune, infective, postpartum, toxic exposure, and so forth
Thyroiditis factitia	↓TSH & ↑fT4 ↑fT3 (sometimes) ↓TG level ↓RAIU	• Caused by ingestion of excessive thyroid hormone • TG levels and RAIU will be decreased
TA & TMNG	↓TSH & ↑fT4 U/S, FNA, RAIU	• Nodules that produce and secrete thyroid hormone independent of TSH stimulation • Insidious onset but similar sequelae as GD • Further evaluation of nodules required due to concerns for cancers, compression, or functional disease • U/S, FNA to characterize the cellularity of the nodules • RAIU: Increased uptake in a patchy distribution

Data from Refs.[1–3,5,10,11,14,16–18,23,28,29]

hormone levels are the primary inhibitor of both TRH and TSH.[13,14] Iodine and iodinated TG in the follicle inhibits thyroid hormone production. Knowledge of this is important in the interpretation of thyroid test results, because various drugs and over-the-counter supplements can alter the levels of TSH and thyroid hormone.[16,17]

PATHOLOGY OF THE THYROID GLAND

Thyroid pathology presents as one of two forms: either a deficit of functional thyroid hormone known as hypothyroidism or an excess of thyroid hormone known as hyperthyroidism. There are three broad mechanisms that cause thyroid pathology: disruption of the structural integrity of the thyroid gland (**Fig. 4**), aberrations in the production of thyroid hormone, or deregulation of thyroid homeostasis at either the HPT or cellular level.[16,18]

Hypothyroidism

Case study 1: carpel tunnel syndrome due to repetitive overuse?

Dan G., a stocker in a grocery chain, presented to the occupational clinic with a history of numbness, tingling, and pain in both wrists. He reported decreased grip strength, worsening over several months. Friends suggested he had carpel tunnel syndrome and needed surgery. On examination, the Physician Assistant (PA) noted a flat affect, goiter, diffuse nonpitting edema, and slowed mentation. Questioning elicited a past medical history of Hashimoto thyroiditis that was initially treated with "some pills," but Dan had stopped taking them.

Hypothyroid disease is a hypometabolic state with low levels of circulating thyroid hormone. It has a heterogeneous presentation and multiple causes. Gravity of the

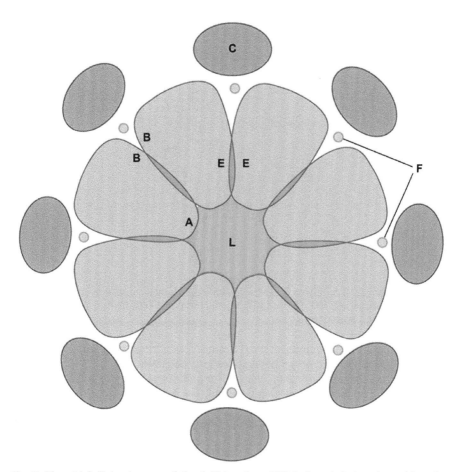

Fig. 2. Thyroid follicle. A, apex of the follicle where TPO is found; B, basolateral junction where TSH stimulates production of thyroid hormone, along with absorption of iodine, and release of thyroid hormone; C, parafollicular or C-Cells where calcitonin is synthesized; E, tight junction between follicular cells; F, fenestrated capillary; L, lumen containing colloid containing iodinated tyrosyl, DIT, MIT, T3, T4.

disease depends on the severity and acuity in which thyroid levels drop below an individual's euthyroid state. Primary hypothyroidism is defined as the inability of the thyroid gland to respond to TSH stimulation. An elevated serum TSH and a low free thyroxine (fT4) confirm the diagnosis.[1,5] Worldwide, iodine deficiency is the most common cause of hypothyroidism. In the United States, Hashimoto thyroiditis is more common (see **Fig. 3**, **Table 3**).[10,17]

Hashimoto thyroiditis, an autoimmune disease, begins with lymphocytic infiltration of the follicle. This infiltration causes inflammation, ensuing follicular destruction, and ultimately, hypothyroidism (see **Fig. 4**). Antibodies associated with Hashimoto thyroiditis include antithyroid peroxidase (TPOAb) and antithyroglobulin antibodies (TGAb).[16,18]

Subacute hypothyroidism is a controversial diagnosis.[19,20] Bojar and colleagues[21] suggest subacute hypothyroidism should be considered when, on 2 separate

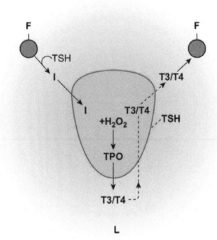

Fig. 3. Follicular cell. F, fenestrated capillary; I, iodine; L, lumen containing colloid containing iodinated tyrosyl, DIT, MIT, T3, T4; T3/T4, thyroid hormone; TPO, thyroid peroxidase; TSH, thyroid stimulating hormone.

occasions, the TSH is elevated, yet the fT4 remains within the reference range. Treatment should be continued only if patients respond positively.

Iatrogenic hypothyroidism occurs when all or part of the thyroid gland is damaged by surgical, chemical or radiologic interventions. The destruction of the thyroid can be intentional or a consequence of treatment of other conditions (see **Table 2**). Treatment is thyroid hormone replacement. Adequacy of replacement is monitored by assessing the TSH level periodically.[1,20]

Congenital hypothyroidism is the most common preventable cause of childhood intellectual impairment. A screening TSH is mandated in all neonates born in the United States.[22,23] Secondary and tertiary hypothyroidism are caused by malfunction of the anterior pituitary or hypothalamus, respectively. In both of these cases, the thyroid gland lacks adequate stimulation to produce thyroid hormone. Treatment and monitoring of thyroid function will vary depending on the primary condition's pathogenesis.[1,17]

Case study 1, continued
A TSH level and fT4 level were obtained with the following results: TSH 125.2 mIU/L (reference range: 0.4–4.8 mIU/L) and fT4 0.5 ng/dL (reference range: 1.0–2.1 ng/dL). Dan was referred to an endocrinologist. Four weeks later, Dan reported significant symptom improvement. His symptoms resolved completely with T4 supplementation. No surgical intervention was needed.

Discussion: Fluid retention is common with hypothyroid disease. In Dan's case, fluid retention and repetitive wrist use precipitated carpel tunnel syndrome. Fluid retention resolved with T4 replacement leading to symptom resolution.

Thyrotoxicosis

Case study 2: iatrogenic thyrotoxicosis
Betty, 56, was diagnosed with primary hyperparathyroidism. Preoperative studies identified a parathyroid adenoma behind the right thyroid lobe. Because Betty

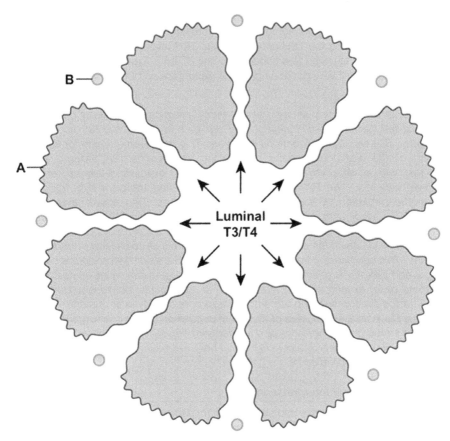

Fig. 4. Folliculitis. A, inflamed follicular cells with disrupted tight junctions; B, fenestrated capillaries.

had osteoporosis, surgical removal of the adenoma was indicated. Surgery and immediate postoperative recovery were uneventful. She went home that evening. Around midnight, Betty developed sweating, anxiety, chest pain, and heart palpitations. She called the answering service and was instructed to go to the Emergency Department by ambulance. She was worked up for a possible heart attack. After testing, the doctor determined Betty had transient hyperthyroidism due to manipulation of her thyroid gland during surgery.

Thyrotoxicosis is a hypermetabolic state with high levels of circulating thyroid hormone from any cause. Hyperthyroidism, by contrast, is an increased production of thyroid hormone by the thyroid gland.[18] The 3 most common causes of hyperthyroidism are Grave disease (GD), toxic adenoma (TA) or a toxic multinodular goiter (TMNG), or by TSH-secreting pituitary tumors (see **Table 3**).[3,16]

GD is a chronic autoimmune disorder in which the body produces TSH-like antibodies that stimulate excessive production and secretion of thyroid hormone. Toxic nodules secrete thyroid hormone independent of TSH stimulation. The onset of symptoms is typically more insidious than GD but can lead to the same sequelae of hyperthyroidism.[16,24]

Thyrotoxicosis can also be caused by increased release of stored thyroid hormone (thyroiditis) or from an extra thyroidal source of thyroid hormone. The morbidity of thyrotoxicosis depends on the severity and acuity in which circulating levels of thyroid hormone increases above euthyroid level. Thyrotoxicosis, regardless of its cause, is confirmed by assessing the TSH and fT4 levels. TSH levels will be very low with an elevated fT4 and/or elevated free triiodothyronine (fT3).[5,17] Treatment and monitoring of thyroid function will vary depending on the pathogenesis of the primary condition.

Case study 2, continued

Three weeks later, Betty was seen at her family practice clinic. Betty complained of severe fatigue and of difficulty getting out of bed and doing her activities of daily living. She was barely functioning at work. This had been ongoing for 2 weeks. As part of the workup for major depressive disorder, her PA ordered a TSH level test with a reflexive fT4 level test. The TSH level was elevated, and the fT4 level was low. The PA determined that Betty had transient hypothyroidism due to the depletion of her stored thyroid hormones. Two weeks later, repeat TSH and fT4 level tests showed normalization of results and resolution of her symptoms.

Discussion: Manipulation of the thyroid gland can cause release of stored thyroid hormone. This can cause a transient thyrotoxicosis. Transient thyrotoxicosis can lead to signs and symptoms of an acute coronary syndrome and can cause acute coronary syndrome or an exacerbation of heart failure in susceptible individuals. Hence, the referral to the Emergency Department was appropriate. However, patient education regarding the potential sequelae of thyroid manipulation during the surgery, with the release of stored thyroid hormone and subsequent depletion, could have saved Betty much in the way of anxiety and concern about her health during her recovery period as well as additional medical costs.

Laboratory Testing and Interpretation

TSH level is the most sensitive and specific test for detecting thyroid dysfunction in the absence of hypothalamic or pituitary disease. It is also the test of choice to monitor thyroid replacement therapy in hypothyroidism.[25] However, any clinical decision to treat hypothyroidism should not be based on a single TSH level. If the TSH level is slightly above reference range or if the fT4 is within normal range, a repeat TSH and fT4 level test should be obtained from the same laboratory after a period of weeks to see if the TSH and fT4 levels have equilibrated. It should also be noted that TSH levels used to diagnose hypothyroidism and TSH levels used to assess thyroid replacement therapy are different.[8]

TSH reference ranges vary depending on the laboratory and methodologies used. Circadian variability of TSH secretion, illness, poorly controlled chronic disease, or medications can also affect laboratory test results.[26] These confounders can make it difficult to determine if inconsistencies between the TSH and fT4 levels are related to thyroid disease or other factors.[3]

TSH testing limitations include inability to detect central hypothyroidism, treated hyperthyroidism, and nonthyroidal illness.[4,26] When results are equivocal, the TSH and fT4 levels should be repeated at least 1 month after the initial levels were drawn and should be redrawn at the same time of day and analyzed using the same methodology. Obtaining and analyzing samples under similar circumstances blunts circadian and methodological variability.[11,21]

According to the American Association of Clinical Endocrinologists, fT4 and fT3 level tests should be ordered only if the clinical picture is unclear. If the TSH is inconclusive, fT4 level is the test of choice for assessing thyroid hormone status.[10] It is also useful in the evaluation of secondary hypothyroidism, prenatal

Table 4	
Nonlaboratory tests	
Fine-needle aspiration (FNA)	• Indicated for definitive diagnosis of benign vs malignant nodules in the thyroid • Usually done with ultrasound guidance • Not usually indicated for cystic nodules or for nodules <1 cm
RAIU	• Uptake pattern helps determine cause of thyroid pathologic condition • Diffuse pattern suggests GD • Solitary nodule uptake suggests a TA • Decreased uptake suggests thyroiditis • "Hot" nodules take up iodine (hyperfunctioning) and are typically noncancerous • "Cold" nodules do not take up iodine (hypofunctioning) and need further workup (FNA)
Ultrasound (U/S)	• U/S, along with TSH, are recommended for evaluation of thyroid nodules ○ Entirely cystic nodules are typically benign ○ Mixed nodules or solid nodules need further workup

Data from Refs.[1–3,16,28,29]

thyroid dysfunction,[19,20] and thyrotoxicosis factitia (see **Table 3**). The Choosing Wisely campaign[27] suggests fT3 has utility in thyrotoxicosis factitia and nonthyroidal illness.[3,28] Thyroid antibodies are typically ordered when autoimmune disease is suspected and assist in developing a treatment plan. TG and calcitonin are less commonly ordered, but are used for diagnosis and monitoring of thyroid cancers.

A discussion of thyroid testing would be incomplete without mentioning imaging studies in the diagnosis of thyroid pathologic condition (**Table 4**). Thyroid ultrasound, along with TSH level testing, is recommended for the evaluation of all thyroid nodules.[29] Radioactive iodine uptake (RAIU) patterns can provide further information about thyroid pathologic condition based on the pattern of iodine uptake.[10] A diffuse uptake pattern supports the diagnosis of GD. Uptake in a "hot" nodule or multiple nodules indicates either a TA or a TMNG, respectively. "Hot" nodules are typically noncancerous, but "cold" or hypofunctioning nodules need further evaluation. An ultrasound-guided fine-needle aspiration can provide a definitive diagnosis of malignant nodules.[29]

REFERENCES

1. Bishop ML, Fody EP, Schoeff LE. Clinical chemistry: principles, techniques, and correlations. 8th edition. Philadelphia: Wolters Kluwer; 2018.
2. American Association for Clinical Chemistry. Thyroid diseases. Available at: https://labtestsonline.org/conditions/thyroid-diseases. Accessed September 9, 2018.
3. Esfandiari NH, Papaleontiou M. Biochemical testing in thyroid disorders. Endocrinol Metab Clin North Am 2017;46:631.
4. Giacomini A MD, Chiesa M, Carraro P. Urgent thyroid-stimulating hormone testing in emergency medicine: a useful tool? J Emerg Med 2015;49:481–7.
5. Stott DJ, Gussekloo J, Kearney PM, et al. Study protocol; thyroid hormone replacement for untreated older adults with subclinical hypothyroidism - a randomized placebo controlled trial (TRUST). BMC Endocr Disord 2017;17:6–17.

6. Zhelev Z, Abbott R, Rogers M, et al. Effectiveness of interventions to reduce ordering of thyroid function tests: a systematic review. BMJ Open 2016;6: e010065.
7. American Thyroid Association. General information/press room. No date. Available at: https://www.thyroid.org/media-main/press-room/. Accessed June 19, 2018.
8. Sheehan MT. Biochemical testing of the thyroid: TSH is the best and, oftentimes, only test needed – a review for primary care. Clin Med Res 2016;14(2):83–92.
9. Ittermann T, Glaser S, Ewert R, et al. Serum thyroid-stimulating hormone levels are not associated with exercise capacity and lung function parameters in two population-based studies. BMC Pulm Med 2014;14:145.
10. Ross DS, Burch HB, Cooper DS, et al. 2016 American Thyroid Association guidelines for diagnosis and management of hyperthyroidism and other causes of thyrotoxicosis. Thyroid 2016;26:1343.
11. Mahadevan S, Sadacharan D, Kannan S, et al. Does time of sampling or food intake alter thyroid function test? Indian J Endocrinol Metab 2017;21:369–72.
12. Matyjaszek-Matuszek B, Pyzik A, Nowakowski A, et al. Diagnostic methods of TSH in thyroid screening tests. Ann Agric Environ Med 2013;20(4):731–5.
13. Mariotti S, Beck-Peccoz P. Physiology of the hypothalamic-pituitary-thyroid axis. In: De Groot LJ, Chrousos G, Dungan K, et al, editors. Endotext [Internet]. South Dartmouth (MA): MDText.com, Inc.; 2016. Available at: https://www.ncbi.nlm.nih.gov/books/NBK278958/.
14. Carvalho DP, Dupuy C. Thyroid hormone biosynthesis and release. Mol Cell Endocrinol 2017;458:6–15.
15. Huang H, Shi Y, Liang B, et al. Iodinated TG in thyroid follicles regulate TSH/TSHR signaling for NIS expression. Biol Trace Elem Res 2017;180:206–13.
16. Merck manual. Thyroid disorders. Available at: https://www.merckmanuals.com/professional/endocrine-and-metabolic-disorders/thyroid-disorders. Accessed December 2, 2018.
17. Garber JR, Cobin RH, Gharib H, et al. Clinical practice guidelines for hypothyroidism in adults: cosponsored by the American Association of Clinical Endocrinologists and the American Thyroid Association. Endocr Pract 2012;18:989.
18. Maitra A. The Endocrine system. In: Kumar V, Abbas AK, Aster JC, et al, editors. Robbins and Cotran pathologic basis of disease. 9th edition. Philadelphia: Elsevier/Saunders; 2015. p. 1073–100.
19. Chan S, Boelaert K. Optimal management of hypothyroidism, hypothyroxinaemia and euthyroid TPO antibody positivity preconception and in pregnancy. Clin Endocrinol 2015;82:313–26.
20. De Groot L, Abalovich M, Alexander EK, et al. Management of thyroid dysfunction during pregnancy and postpartum: an Endocrine Society clinical practice guideline. J Clin Endocrinol Metab 2012;97:2543–65.
21. Bojar I, Bejga P, Witczak M, et al. Standards for thyroid laboratory testing, and cognitive functions after menopause. Prz Menopauzalny 2014;13:233–41.
22. Singh RJ, Kaur P. Thyroid hormone testing in the 21st century. Clin Biochem 2016; 49:843–5.
23. Underland L, Kenigsberg L, Derrick KM, et al. Thyroid function testing in neonates with maternal history of disease. Clin Pediatr 2018;57:436–41.
24. Durante C, Grani G, Lamartina L, et al. The diagnosis and management of thyroid nodules: a review. JAMA 2018;319:914–24.
25. Gill J, Barakauskas VE, Thomas D, et al. Evaluation of thyroid test utilization through analysis of population-level data. Clin Chem Lab Med 2017;55:1898.

26. Golombek SG. nonthyroidal illness syndrome and euthyroid sick syndrome in intensive care patients. Semin Perinatol 2008;32:413–8.
27. Choosing wisely: Endocrine Society and American Association of Clinical Endocrinologists, five things physicians and patients should question. Choosing Wisely, initiative of the ABIM Foundation Website. Available at: https://www.choosingwisely.org/clinician-lists/endocrine-society-total-or-free-t3-level-when-assessing-levothryroxine-dose-in-hyperthyroid-patients/. Accessed December 31, 2018.
28. Kluesner J, Beckman D, Tate J, et al. Analysis of current thyroid function test ordering practices. J Eval Clin Pract 2018;24:347–52.
29. Roth MY, Witt RL, Steward DL. Molecular testing for thyroid nodules: review and current state: molecular testing for thyroid nodules. Cancer 2018;124:888–98.

Hepatic Function Testing
The ABCs of the Liver Function Tests

M. Jane McDaniel, MS, MLS(ASCP)SC

KEYWORDS

- Hepatic function tests • Bilirubin metabolism • Hepatocellular injury • Cholestasis
- Prehepatic jaundice • Hepatic jaundice • Posthepatic jaundice

KEY POINTS

- Understanding the physiology behind the bilirubin pathway and the pathophysiology resulting from disruptions in the normal pathway can assist in evaluating hepatic function test results.
- Fractionated bilirubin, aspartate aminotransferase, alanine aminotransferase, alkaline phosphatase, and γ-glutamyl transferase are the major hepatic function tests used to differentiate between prehepatic, hepatic, and posthepatic jaundice.
- Evaluation of a patient with jaundice requires a detailed history and focused laboratory evaluation.

INTRODUCTION

Hepatobiliary injury or disease is a common entity investigated by clinicians and begins with assessment of any abnormal hepatic function tests. Hepatobiliary injury or disease typically presents with varying degrees of elevation of serum bilirubin (total, conjugated, and/or unconjugated), serum aspartate aminotransferase (AST), serum alanine aminotransferase (ALT), serum alkaline phosphatase (ALP), and/or serum γ-glutamyl transferase (GGT). Evaluation of the pattern of elevations in these hepatic function tests can assist the clinician in determining if a patient has prehepatic, hepatic, or posthepatic organ involvement in the injury or disease process.

PHYSIOLOGY OF THE BILIRUBIN PATHWAY

To better understand the various components of total bilirubin, it is important to understand the biochemical pathways for bilirubin production and excretion (**Fig. 1**). Most bilirubin is produced by the breakdown of hemoglobin to indirect (unconjugated) bilirubin, which is not water soluble. In order to be transported in the circulation, indirect (unconjugated) bilirubin is bound to albumin. The indirect (unconjugated) bilirubin/albumin complex is carried to the liver, where the conversion of indirect (unconjugated)

Disclosure Statement: Nothing to disclose.
Yale Physician Assistant Online Program, Yale School of Medicine, 100 Church Street South, Suite A230, New Haven, CT 06519, USA
E-mail address: jane.mcdaniel@yale.edu

Physician Assist Clin 4 (2019) 541–550
https://doi.org/10.1016/j.cpha.2019.02.013
2405-7991/19/© 2019 Elsevier Inc. All rights reserved.

physicianassistant.theclinics.com

Normal Bilirubin Pathway

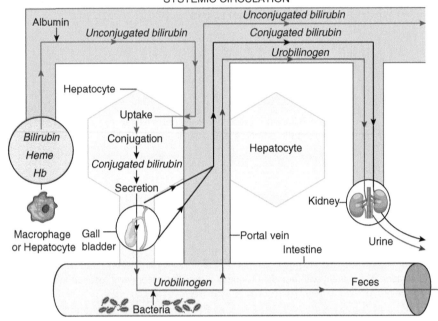

Fig. 1. Normal bilirubin pathway.

bilirubin to direct (conjugated) bilirubin occurs via the covalent linkage of the indirect (unconjugated) bilirubin to glucuronic acid by the enzyme glucuronyl transferase. This creates direct (conjugated) bilirubin, which is water soluble and can be excreted in the bile.[1] The majority of direct (conjugated) bilirubin is excreted via the biliary system into the gut, where bacteria break down the direct (conjugated) bilirubin into urobilinogen. Urobilinogen in the gut is (1) reabsorbed from the intestine and carried by the portal circulation back to the liver to be recirculated in the bile, (2) reabsorbed from the intestine and carried by the systemic circulation to the kidneys and excreted in the urine, or (3) converted to stercobilin (which gives feces its brown color) and excreted in the feces. In a patient with normal breakdown of hemoglobin and normal hepatic and biliary function, the total serum bilirubin is less than or equal to 1.0 mg/dL, with indirect (unconjugated) bilirubin comprising approximately 70% of the total serum bilirubin.[2]

PATHOPHYSIOLOGY: PREHEPATIC JAUNDICE

Prehepatic conditions result in an increase in only indirect (unconjugated) bilirubin in the blood. In these instances, there is an increase in the breakdown of hemoglobin, causing an increased amount of indirect (unconjugated) bilirubin in the blood. Patients with only increased indirect (unconjugated) bilirubin (>70% of the total bilirubin value) typically do not have serious liver disease. Rather, the liver's ability to conjugate and excrete bilirubin is overwhelmed, resulting in increased levels of indirect (unconjugated) bilirubin and, therefore, increased levels of total serum bilirubin (although rarely >5 mg/dL). Increases in indirect (unconjugated) bilirubin exclusively most commonly are seen in increased destruction of erythrocytes (hemolysis), Gilbert syndrome (an inherited benign trait seen in 3%–5% of the population), or Crigler-Najjar syndrome (a rare inherited disorder) or as a result of various drug toxicities[1] (Fig. 2).

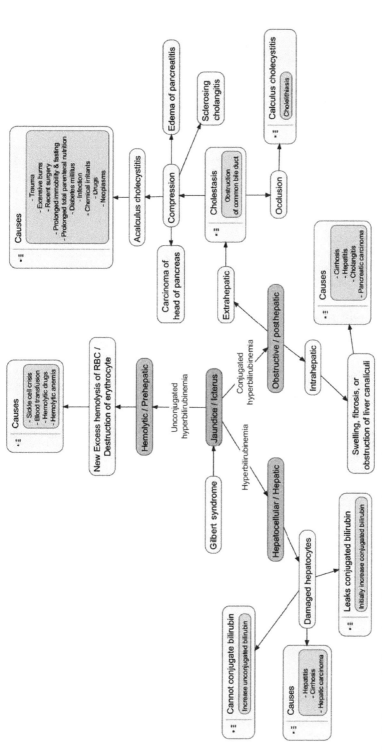

Fig. 2. Prehepatic, hepatic, and posthepatic jaundice: mechanisms and causes. (*From* Wikipedia. Available at: https://en.wikipedia.org/wiki/File: Jaundice-types.png.)

Table 1
Laboratory findings in abnormal bilirubin pathways

	Laboratory Findings
Prehepatic jaundice	↑ indirect (unconjugated) bilirubin in serum ↑ urobilinogen in urine and feces
Hepatic jaundice	↑ indirect (unconjugated) bilirubin in serum ↑ direct (conjugated) bilirubin in serum (if liver still conjugating) ↓ direct (conjugated) bilirubin in gut resulting in: pale stools, bile in urine, no urobilinogen in urine
Posthepatic jaundice	↑ direct (conjugated) bilirubin in serum ↓ direct (conjugated) bilirubin in gut resulting in: pale stools, bile in urine, no urobilinogen in urine

In addition to the increased indirect (unconjugated) bilirubin and the normal direct (conjugated) bilirubin in the serum, there also is an increased direct (conjugated) bilirubin in the gut and increased urobilinogen in the urine and feces due to the increased breakdown of indirect (unconjugated) bilirubin by the liver (**Table 1**).

PATHOPHYSIOLOGY: HEPATIC JAUNDICE

Injury or disease of the liver results in increases in both indirect (unconjugated) and direct (conjugated) bilirubin in the blood and is caused by injured hepatocytes, which impairs the uptake of indirect (unconjugated) bilirubin, the conjugation of indirect (unconjugated) bilirubin to direct (conjugated) bilirubin, and/or the excretion of direct (conjugated) bilirubin into the bile ducts.[3] Patients with hepatic injury or disease have elevated levels of indirect (unconjugated) bilirubin in the serum due to impaired functioning of the hepatocytes, which results in the reduced ability to form direct (conjugated) bilirubin, and elevated levels of direct (conjugated) bilirubin due to the swollen hepatic ducts which block excretion of any direct (conjugated) bilirubin that is formed by the hepatocytes. Although the total bilirubin consists of both indirect (unconjugated) and direct (conjugated) bilirubin, the direct (conjugated) bilirubin constitutes greater than 50% of the total bilirubin. The primary causes of increased direct (unconjugated) bilirubin are hepatitis, cirrhosis, and hepatic carcinoma (see **Fig. 2**). Two rare inherited conditions that are also associated with an elevated direct (conjugated) bilirubin are Dubin-Johnson syndrome and Rotor syndrome, where direct (conjugated) bilirubin in the blood is elevated with all other liver function tests being normal.[2] In addition to increased indirect (unconjugated) and direct (conjugated) bilirubin in the serum, hepatic jaundice also causes decreased direct (conjugated) bilirubin in the gut, resulting in pale stools and no urobilinogen in the urine, because there is no direct (conjugated) bilirubin to break down into urobilinogen and stercobilin. Direct (conjugated) bilirubin is excreted in the urine by the kidneys due to direct (conjugated) bilirubin present in the serum (see **Table 1**). Direct (conjugated) bilirubin in the urine is never a normal finding.

PATHOPHYSIOLOGY: POSTHEPATIC JAUNDICE

Posthepatic jaundice results in an increase in only direct (conjugated) bilirubin in the blood and is caused by obstruction in the bile ducts, which blocks excretion of direct (conjugated) bilirubin into the gut, including

- Intrahepatic obstruction due to functional impairments of bile formation by the hepatocytes,[2] such as tumors, cholestasis, cholangitis, pancreatic carcinoma, or other obstructions blocking the excretion of direct (conjugated) bilirubin from the liver
- Extrahepatic obstruction due to anatomic obstructions to bile flow,[2] such as tumors, gallstones (cholelithiasis), obstruction of the common bile duct (cholestasis), or any of the other mechanisms listed in **Fig. 2**

Although direct (conjugated) bilirubin levels are increased in intrahepatic jaundice, levels of direct (conjugated) bilirubin tend to be even higher in extrahepatic jaundice.[4] As in hepatic jaundice, the direct (conjugated) bilirubin in the blood constitutes greater than 50% of the total bilirubin. In addition to increased direct (conjugated) bilirubin in the serum, posthepatic jaundice also causes decreased direct (conjugated) bilirubin in the gut, resulting in pale stools and no urobilinogen in the urine (no direct bilirubin to break down into urobilinogen and stercobilin) as well as the presence of bilirubin in the urine (which is never normal). Bilirubin in the urine is due to direct (conjugated) bilirubin present in the serum and excreted by the kidneys (see **Table 1**).

BILIRUBIN SUMMARY

Elevated direct (conjugated) bilirubin is found in both cholestasis and hepatocellular liver disease. In particular, bilirubin levels can serve as a marker of liver disease severity, because elevated levels of direct (conjugated) bilirubin are not found in blood until more than 50% of the liver's excretory capacity is lost.[5] In addition, there is a gray area that exists between indirect (unconjugated) and direct (conjugated) hyperbilirubinemia. Typically, if greater than 50% of the total bilirubin is composed of direct (conjugated) bilirubin, the diagnosis points to either hepatic or posthepatic jaundice, whereas if less than 30% of the total bilirubin is composed of direct (conjugated) bilirubin, the diagnosis points to prehepatic jaundice. If the fraction of direct (conjugated) bilirubin falls between 30% and 50%, other liver function and hematologic tests may be required to determine the cause of the jaundice.[1] In addition, a thorough history (in particular, for exposure to drugs, alcohol, and toxins), physical examination, and additional laboratory studies are critical in determining the exact cause of elevated bilirubin levels. Once the cause of the (direct) conjugated hyperbilirubinemia has resolved, bilirubin levels decreases in a bimodal fashion with rapid metabolism of free bilirubin occurring first. This is followed by a slower decrease in direct (conjugated) bilirubin that is bound to albumin, termed delta bilirubin. Delta bilirubin has the same half-life as albumin and is, therefore, metabolized at a much slower rate.[6]

HEPATIC FUNCTION TESTS: AMINOTRANSFERASES

The aminotransferases most often are associated with hepatocellular damage and consist of AST and ALT. AST is found in heart, liver, skeletal muscle, and kidney cells, whereas ALT is found primarily in the liver. Therefore, an increase in AST without concomitant increase in ALT may suggest cardiac or muscle disease rather than liver disease. These enzymes are located inside hepatocytes and are important in various metabolic pathways. When there is hepatocellular injury, ALT and AST are released into the serum in greater quantities than other hepatic enzymes and are sensitive markers for hepatocyte damage[2] (**Table 2**).

ALT is found in the cytoplasm of the hepatocytes, is the first enzyme to be released in hepatocellular injury, and is more elevated in acute conditions. AST is found in the cytoplasm and mitochondria of the hepatocytes, and its release into the serum

Table 2
Relationship of aspartate aminotransferase and alanine aminotransferase to alkaline phosphatase and γ-glutamyl transferase in liver diseases

Liver Disease	Aspartate Amino-transferase	Alanine Aminotransferase	Aspartate Aminotransferase/ Alanine Aminotransferase	Alkaline Phosphatase	γ-Glutamyl Transferase
Acute hepatitis	↑ 10×–20×	↑ 10×–30×	<1.0	N to ↑ 3×	N to ↑ 3×
Chronic hepatitis	N to ↑ 10×	N to ↑ 8×	<2.0	N to ↑ 3×	N to ↑ 3×
Alcoholic liver disease	N to ↑ 10×	N to ↑ 2×	>2.0	N to ↑ 3×	↑ 1×–10×
Intrahepatic cholestasis	↑ 1×–5×	N to ↑ 3×	>1.5	N to ↑ 7×	N to ↑ 7×
Extrahepatic cholestasis	N to ↑ 3×	N to ↑ 4×	<1.5	↑ 2×–10×	↑ 1×–10×
Malignancy	N to ↑ 4×	N to ↑ 3×	>1.5	↑ 2×–12×	↑ 1×–7×

Data from Refs.[2,6,8,13]

typically is delayed, resulting in a greater prevalence in chronic conditions. This variation in the release of ALT and AST can be used to distinguish clinical conditions by calculating the ratio of AST to ALT, also known as the De Ritis ratio. In addition to the magnitude of AST and ALT elevations, the De Ritis ratio can help determine the etiology of abnormal aminotransferase results.[7] For example, the AST/ALT ratio in acute viral hepatitis typically is less than 1.0, because ALT is released more rapidly than AST. In chronic hepatitis, however, greater quantities of AST are released and the ratio can become greater than1.0 but less than 2.0. The ratio is occasionally elevated in patients with nonalcoholic steatohepatitis (NAHS) and patients with hepatitis C who have developed cirrhosis, although the ratio typically is not greater than 2.0. Alcoholic liver disease, such as hepatic steatosis, hepatitis, and cirrhosis, is associated with a ratio of greater than or equal to 2.0 with AST values rarely exceeding 300 IU/dL.[8] **Table 2** outlines the expected De Ritis ratio values seen in specific disease entities.

HEPATIC FUNCTION TESTS: ALKALINE PHOSPHATASE AND γ-GLUTAMYL TRANSFERASE

ALP is an enzyme found in bone, liver, intestine, kidney, leukocytes, and placenta. It is one of the first enzymes elevated in cholestatic liver diseases, which can be categorized as anatomic obstructions to bile flow (extrahepatic cholestasis) or as functional impairments of bile formation by the hepatocytes (intrahepatic cholestasis). Because ALP elevations can be due to nonhepatic sources, it is important to differentiate hepatic ALP from nonhepatic sources. If ALP is elevated in the presence of other elevated liver chemistries, it may not be necessary to confirm that the ALP is of hepatic origin. If the ALP elevation is isolated, however, confirmation with GGT or 5'-nucleotidase can help determine if the ALP elevation is hepatic in origin.[2]

GGT is the most sensitive enzyme in liver disease but has a low specificity, because it can also be elevated in patients with pancreatic disease, myocardial infarction, renal failure, emphysema, and diabetes and with patients on certain medications (phenytoin and barbiturates).[2,9,10] If the GGT is normal, however, hepatic involvement is not necessarily excluded, because ALP and GGT do not always rise together in liver disease. GGT is particularly sensitive to alcohol ingestion, because alcohol induces the synthesis of GGT. In cases of a question that the GGT elevation may be due to alcohol, it GGT levels do not return to normal until 3 weeks to 5 weeks after cessation of alcohol consumption.[4] Another enzyme that can aid in determining if ALP elevation is hepatic in origin is 5′-nucelotidase, which was found slightly more specific for correlation to hepatic involvement than GGT.[11]

Once the ALP elevation has been confirmed as hepatic in origin, the presence of symptoms and patient history are important factors for determining specific disease entities.[6] Some of these disease entities and the clinical presentations they are associated with include

- Biliary obstruction: right upper quandrant pain and fever
- Cholestatic drug reactions: medications suspected in the presence of increased bilirubin and/or AST and ALT
- Primary biliary cirrhosis: women with other autoimmune diseases
- Primary sclerosing cholangitis: inflammatory bowel disease

In addition, extrahepatic malignancies also can present with elevated ALP and GGT levels.[6]

Table 2 outlines the expected elevations of AST, ALT, ALP, and GGT found in specific disease states. Elevated aminotransferase levels also may result from hepatic infiltration from metastatic or primary hepatocellular carcinoma, tuberculosis, sarcoidosis, and amyloidosis, causing modest increases (as much as 3-times normal) in aminotransferase levels and as much as 20-fold increases in ALP with typically normal bilirubin levels.[12]

LIVER INJURY ASSESSMENT USING *R* RATIO

The American College of Gastroenterology clinical guidelines published in 2014 and 2017 describe the use of an *R* ratio to assess the pattern of liver injury. This ratio can be used to determine whether the injury is hepatocellular, cholestatic, or mixed and is calculated using the following formula:

R = (ALT value/ALT upper limit of normal)/(ALP value/ALP upper limit of normal)

An *R* ratio of greater than 5 identifies the liver injury as hepatocellular, whereas an *R* ratio of less than 2 identifies the liver injury as cholestatic, and an *R* ratio between 2 and 5 indicates a mixed pattern.[2,14]

NONHEPATIC TESTS FOR ASSESSMENT OF LIVER FUNCTION

Several laboratory tests that are not routinely considered to be hepatic function tests can be strong indicators in the assessment of hepatic synthetic function. Albumin is a plasma protein that is synthesized exclusively in the liver and has a half-life of 14 days to 21 days.[5] Serum albumin is not a good marker of acute liver dysfunction, because it can be normal in acute liver disease. Serum albumin may be decreased, however, in chronic liver disease. Low serum albumin can be the result of many nonhepatic causes and is not appropriate for use to assess liver function if hepatic function tests are normal.

Clotting factors also are synthesized exclusively in the liver, with the exception of factor VIII. Factor VII has the shortest half-life (6 hours) of all the clotting factors and, therefore, is a good estimate of acute changes in the liver's synthetic capabilities. Factor VII can be assessed using prothrombin time (PT), and PT is not prolonged until the concentration of factor VII falls below 10% of normal.[15] Consequently, prolonged PT can be useful in assessing the severity of acute liver disease.

HEPATIC FUNCTION TESTS IN LIVER DISEASE
Acute Hepatitis

Acute hepatitis is characterized by the presence of jaundice or nonspecific symptoms of acute illness accompanied by increased levels of AST and ALT, with the De Ritis ratio less than 1.0, and greater than 50% of total bilirubin is accounted for by direct (conjugated) bilirubin. AST and ALT elevations of greater than 10-times normal are seen in acute hepatic injury and are seldom that high in other liver diseases. ALP in these patients is typically less than 3 times the upper reference limit.[16] In addition to hepatic function tests, testing should be initiated for antigens and antibodies to hepatitis A, hepatitis B, and hepatitis C. Evaluation of these testing modalities, however, is not within the scope of this article. Acute viral hepatitis A and hepatitis B are typically self-limited, with occasional conversion of hepatitis B to a chronic hepatitis. There currently is no test to definitively diagnose acute hepatitis C because both antigens and antibodies to hepatitis C can be present in both acute and chronic hepatitis C infections.[16] Testing for hepatitis D should be limited to patients who are positive for hepatitis B and have an atypical clinical course, and testing for hepatitis E should be limited to patients who have recently traveled to endemic areas.

Chronic Hepatitis

Chronic hepatitis is defined as ongoing hepatic necrosis and inflammation of the liver, is often accompanied by fibrosis, may progress to cirrhosis, and predisposes the patient to hepatocellular carcinoma.[16] It is determined by the presence of an increased ALT for greater than 6 months after an episode of acute hepatitis or increased ALT on more than one occasion over a period of 6 months. Chronic hepatitis most commonly is the result of chronic viral infection, typically hepatitis C.[16] In chronic hepatitis, AST and ALT elevations are seen but not to the same degree as seen in acute hepatitis, and the De Ritis ratio typically is less than 1.0 and can be elevated above 1.0 in severe cases but not above 2.0 unless a patient has chronic alcoholic hepatitis. As in acute hepatitis, greater than 50% of total bilirubin is accounted for by direct (conjugated) bilirubin in chronic hepatitis.

Alcoholic Hepatitis

Alcoholic hepatitis usually occurs after months or years of heavy alcohol use. Clinical symptoms include jaundice, right upper quadrant pain, fever, and anorexia. If clinical history suggests alcohol abuse and if ALT is substantially higher than the AST, the most probable diagnosis is alcoholic hepatitis.[16] Additional laboratory findings include an elevated total bilirubin with the direct (conjugated) bilirubin greater than 50% of the total, an extremely elevated GGT (up to 10-times normal), moderately elevated AST and ALT, and a De Ritis ratio of greater than 2.0 (and sometimes >5.0).

Hepatic Steatosis and Nonalcoholic Steatohepatitis

Nonalcoholic fatty liver disease is the most common cause of asymptomatic elevation of transaminase levels and is divided into 2 subtypes, nonalcoholic fatty liver (hepatic steatosis without inflammation) and NASH, which includes hepatocyte injury and inflammation and can lead to fibrosis. Patients with NASH have a high risk of progression to cirrhosis and hepatocellular carcinoma.[17] Patients with NASH typically have mildly elevated AST and ALT (usually less than 4-times normal), with a De Ritis ratio that is usually less than 1.0.[18] Changes in the liver can be seen on ultrasound or MRI for both types of nonalcoholic fatty liver disease, but the only way to confirm a diagnosis of NASH is with a biopsy.

Cirrhosis

The classification of chronic hepatitis is based on inflammatory activity and degree of fibrosis. Although biopsy is the only definitive marker of progression from chronic hepatitis to cirrhosis, markers of hepatic function may be an initial indicator.[16] Specific markers of hepatic function found in progression to cirrhosis include increased AST and ALT, with a De Ritis ratio (AST/ALT) often less than 1.0 in early cirrhosis and greater than 1.0 in late cirrhosis, decreased albumin, increased PT/international normalized ratio, decreased platelet count, and (in late cirrhosis) hyponatremia. As cirrhosis progresses and fibrosis increases, the De Ritis ratio (AST/ALT) increases, which can be attributed to the reduced production of ALT in the damaged liver.[16]

SUMMARY

The evaluation of a patient with suspected hepatobiliary injury or disease should begin with a detailed history and an assessment of any abnormal hepatic function tests. Hepatobiliary injury or disease typically presents with varying degrees of elevation of bilirubin, either total, direct (conjugated), and/or indirect (unconjugated). Further diagnostic studies to be considered include serum AST, serum ALT, serum ALP, and serum GGT. Patterns of elevation in these hepatic function tests can assist the clinician in determining if a patient has prehepatic, hepatic, or posthepatic organ involvement and can lead to the diagnosis of many liver and biliary diseases.

REFERENCES

1. Farkas P, Sampson J, Slitzky B, et al. Liver and gastroenterology tests. In: Lee M, editor. Basic skills in interpreting laboratory data. 6th edition. Bethesda (MD): American Society of Health-System Pharmacists; 2017. p. 329–68.
2. Kwo PY, Cohen SM, Lim JK. ACG clinical guideline: evaluation of abnormal liver chemistries. Am J Gastroenterol 2017;112:18–35.
3. Woreta TA, Alqahtani SA. Evaluation of abnormal liver tests. Med Clin North Am 2014;98(1):1–16.
4. Sacher RA, McPherson RA. Widmann's clinical interpretation of laboratory tests. 11th edition. Philadelphia: F A Davis Company; 2000. p. 562–99.
5. Agrawal S, Dhiman RK, Limdi JK. Evaluation of abnormal liver function tests. Postgrad Med J 2016;92:223–34.
6. Giannini EG, Testa R, Savarino V. Liver enzyme alteration: a guide for clinicians. CMAJ 2005;172(3):367–79.
7. Botros M, Sikaris KA. The De Ritis ratio: the test of time. Clin Biochem Rev 2013; 34:117–30.
8. Green RM, Flamm S. AGA technical review on the evaluation of liver chemistry tests. Gastroenterology 2002;123:1367–84.
9. Kim HW, Lee SH, Lee DH. Relationship of serum gamma-glutamyltransferase levels with pulmonary function and chronic obstructive pulmonary disease. Lung 2014;192:719–27.
10. Lum G, Gambino SR. Serum gamma-glutamyl transpeptidase activity as an indicator of disease of liver, pancreas, or bone. Clin Chem 1972;18:358–62.

11. Waalkes TP, Abeloff MD, Ettinger DS, et al. Biological markers as an aid in the clinical management of patients with liver metastases. J Surg Oncol 1982; 20(2):83–94.

12. Limdi JK, Hyde GM. Evaluation of abnormal liver function tests. Postgrad Med J 2003;79:307–12.

13. McClatchey KD. Clinical laboratory medicine. Williams & Wilkins: Baltimore (MD); 1994.

14. Chalasani NP, Hayashi PH, Bonkovsky HL, et al. ACG clinical guideline: the diagnosis and management of idiosyncratic drug-induced liver injury. Am J Gastroenterol 2014;109:950–66.

15. Dufour DR, Lott JA, Nolte FS, et al. Diagnosis and monitoring of hepatic injury. I. Performance characteristics of laboratory tests. Clin Chem 2000;46:2027–49.

16. Dufour DR, Lott JA, Nolte FS, et al. Diagnosis and monitoring of hepatic injury. II. Recommendations for use of laboratory tests in screening, diagnosis and monitoring. Clin Chem 2000;46:2050–68.

17. Oh RC, Hustead TR, Ali SM, et al. Mildly elevated liver transaminase levels: causes and evaluation. Am Fam Physician 2017;96(11):709–15.

18. Pratt DS, Kaplan MM. Evaluation of abnormal liver-enzyme results in asymptomatic patients. N Engl J Med 2000;342(17):1266–71.

Arterial Blood Gas Interpretation Demystified

Debra A. Herrmann, DHSc, MPH, PA-C

KEYWORDS

- ABG interpretation • ABG analysis • Arterial blood gases • Acid-base balance

KEY POINTS

- The body's regulation of pH is influenced by both the respiratory and the metabolic systems, where bicarbonate represents the metabolic influence, and partial pressure of carbon dioxide represents the respiratory influence.
- pH is dependent on the ratio of partial pressure of carbon dioxide to bicarbonate. A change in partial pressure of carbon dioxide is compensated by a change in bicarbonate and vice versa.
- Respiratory compensation in metabolic acid-base disorders is fast and activated within minutes; metabolic compensation in respiratory acid-base disorders is slow, with activation taking hours to days.
- An anion gap calculation (corrected for low albumin if necessary) is essential for analyzing an arterial blood gas test correctly.
- Physician assistants need a systematic approach to arterial blood gas interpretation to increase accuracy and confidence in this foundational clinical skill.

Arterial blood gas (ABG) analysis is a routine laboratory test used to assess a patient's oxygenation status and acid-base balance.[1] Physician assistants (PAs) caring for critically ill patients will want to order an ABG to

- Identify and monitor problems with gas exchange and ventilation
- Monitor gas exchange and ventilation in response to interventions or therapy
- Identify and monitor acid-base disturbances
- Assess the response to therapeutic interventions for acid-base disorders[1–3]

ABG analysis is also used in the detection and quantification of levels of abnormal hemoglobins (eg, carboxyhemoglobin and methemoglobin)[2,3]; however, that indication for an ABG analysis is not discussed in this review.

The specimen for ABG analysis is arterial blood because arterial blood (rather than venous blood) is the best indicator of how well the lungs are oxygenating.[4] Arterial

Disclosure Statement: No disclosures.
Department of Physician Assistant Studies, The George Washington University, 2100 Pennsylvania Avenue, Northwest, Suite 300, Washington, DC 20037, USA
E-mail address: dee2a@gwu.edu

Physician Assist Clin 4 (2019) 551–560
https://doi.org/10.1016/j.cpha.2019.02.008
2405-7991/19/© 2019 Elsevier Inc. All rights reserved.

blood can be collected by a percutaneous needle puncture of an artery or from an indwelling arterial catheter.[2,3] The most common site for percutaneous needle puncture collection is the radial artery because it is accessible, is easily palpated, and has a good collateral supply (something that must be ensured using the Modified Allen test before specimen collection).[2-4]

An ABG analysis includes a measurement of the concentration of following substances found in arterial blood[2]:

- The partial pressure of oxygen (Pao_2)
- The partial pressure of carbon dioxide ($Paco_2$)
- Acidity (pH)
- Oxyhemoglobin saturation (SaO_2)
- Bicarbonate (HCO_3)

Unlike other laboratory tests for which it is essential to evaluate each test of a panel separately, ABG results need to be interpreted as 1 result.[4] **Table 1** shows normal values for components of the ABG analysis.

This article seeks to demystify ABG analysis to allow PAs to rapidly, accurately, and confidently interpret ABGs using a systematic method. To accomplish this goal, a review of the relevant acid-base physiology is presented followed by an outline of a stepwise approach that can be applied to 3 case studies.

ACID-BASE PHYSIOLOGY

The correct interpretation of an ABG analysis is not possible without an understanding of the underlying physiology of acid-base balance in the body. A patient's acid-base balance is measured by the hydrogen ion (H^+) concentration in the blood (pH).[5] Bodily functions are optimized in a blood pH range of 7.35 to 7.45, and neutral blood pH is 7.4.[4] A blood pH less than 7.35 is called acidemia, whereas a pH greater than 7.45 is considered alkalemia.[6] Various processes in the body, such as respiratory/metabolic acidosis and respiratory/metabolic alkalosis, result in changes in the blood pH, thereby resulting in acidemia or alkalemia.[6]

Both the respiratory and the metabolic systems influence the body's regulation of pH. The Henderson-Hasselbalch equation[6] reveals the mathematical relationship between pH, HCO_3, and $Paco_2$:

$$pH = 6.1 + \log\left[\frac{HCO_3}{PaCO_2 \times 0.03}\right]$$

In this equation, HCO_3 represents the metabolic influence on pH, whereas $Paco_2$ represents the respiratory influence on blood pH. The following text reviews the

Table 1	
Normal components of arterial blood gas test results	
Element	**Normal Range**
Acidity (pH)	7.35–7.45
Oxyhemoglobin saturation (SaO_2)	80%–100%
Partial pressure of oxygen (Pao_2)	80–100 mm Hg
Partial pressure of carbon dioxide ($Paco_2$)	35–45 mm Hg
Bicarbonate (HCO_3)	22–27 mEq/L

Data from Larkin BG, Zimmanck RJ. Interpreting arterial blood gases successfully. AORN J 2015;102(4):343–57.

primary and compensatory influences of the respiratory and metabolic systems on acid-base balance.

The Respiratory System's Primary Influence on pH

Carbon dioxide (CO_2) is a normal by-product of cellular metabolism that is carried in the blood to the lungs for removal; therefore, $Paco_2$ in arterial blood is controlled by the lungs through the process of ventilation.[4] In respiratory acidosis, as the $Paco_2$ increases in the blood, the blood pH decreases (causing acidemia). In respiratory alkalosis, the $Paco_2$ in arterial blood decreases and the blood pH increases (causing alkalemia). The relationship between $Paco_2$ and pH can be visualized as a see-saw (see Figure 1 at ref#).[4]

A clinical example of alkalemia caused by a decrease of $Paco_2$ can be seen in patients who are hyperventilating. These patients blow off (or rid the body of) CO_2 (a respiratory acid), thereby developing an alkalemia.[7] A clinical example of acidemia caused by a respiratory condition can be seen in patients with chronic obstructive pulmonary disease (COPD). In COPD, CO_2 (a respiratory acid) is retained because of obstruction and hypoventilation. Carbon dioxide retention raises the $Paco_2$, resulting in an acidemia.[7]

The Respiratory System's Compensatory Influence on pH

When metabolic acidosis or alkalosis disorders are present, the body tries to restore acid-base balance through respiratory compensatory mechanisms. Respiratory compensation in metabolic acid-base disorders is fast and activated within minutes.[3,6] As blood pH decreases due to metabolic acidosis, ventilation increases, causing a subsequent decrease of $Paco_2$, thereby attempting to restore the $Paco_2$/HCO_3 ratio (and pH) toward the normal range.[4,8] As the blood pH increases from a metabolic alkalosis, the respiratory compensation is decreased ventilation, resulting in a secondary increase in $Paco_2$; as stated above, this attempts to restore the $Paco_2$/HCO_3 balance, which shifts the pH toward the normal range.[4,8]

The Metabolic System's Primary Influence on pH

As mentioned above, HCO_3 is the metabolic influence on pH and is considered a base. The kidneys primarily regulate the amount of HCO_3 in the body.[4] The HCO_3 and pH relationship can be visualized as an elevator (see Figure 2 at ref#).[4] As HCO_3 increases in the blood, the pH increases, causing an alkalemia; a decrease in HCO_3 in the blood results in a reduction of the pH, causing an acidemia. Severe prolonged diarrhea causes excessive loss of HCO_3 (a metabolic base), resulting in acidemia.[7] Conversely, prolonged vomiting causes excessive loss of H^+ ions from the gastrointestinal tract, resulting in an imbalance of acid (H^+ ions) and base (HCO_3) circulating in the blood, leading to an alkalemia.[7]

The Metabolic System's Compensatory Influence on pH

There are metabolic compensatory mechanisms to restore acid-base balance in the body due to respiratory acidosis or respiratory alkalosis. As blood pH decreases (due to respiratory acidosis), the kidneys retain HCO_3. When blood pH increases (due to respiratory alkalosis), the kidneys excrete HCO_3 in urine.[4] Unlike respiratory compensation, metabolic compensatory mechanisms are slow and take hours to days to get activated.[4,6]

Putting It All Together: A Summary of Acid-Base Control

Returning to the Henderson-Hasselbalch equation, when considering both the primary and the compensatory influences of the respiratory and metabolic systems, one can conclude that pH is dependent on the $Paco_2$/HCO_3 ratio, and therefore, a change in

$Paco_2$ is compensated by a shift in HCO_3 and vice versa.[4] This fact is foundational to understanding the difference between a primary acid-base disorder with appropriate compensation versus mixed acid-base disorders. A quick way to determine if there is a single (primary) or mixed (complex) acid-base disorder is to consider the following:

- In a primary acid-base disorder, the $Paco_2$ and HCO_3 move in the same direction (ie, both the CO_2 and the HCO_3 are increased).
- In a mixed acid-base disorder, the $Paco_2$ and HCO_3 move in the opposite direction (ie, the CO_2 is increased, whereas the HCO_3 is decreased).[4]

ARTERIAL BLOOD GAS INTERPRETATION

Several methods are used in clinical practice for ABG interpretation, including stepwise approaches, tables, figures, case studies, illustrations, computer-based learning modules, and a tic-tac-toe approach.[7] PAs should determine the method that works best for their particular learning style and that leads to an accurate ABG analysis.[7] For this review, a stepwise approach combining and adapting different strategies[4,6,8–10] from other stepwise approaches was developed and is outlined in **Table 2**.

Step 1: Gather All the Necessary Data

The first step involves ordering an ABG and basic metabolic panel (BMP) on the patient. It is imperative that these blood samples (arterial for the ABG and venous for the BMP) be collected and sent for laboratory analysis at the same time. The PA must then ensure that the HCO_3 results from the BMP (sometimes reported as CO_2 on the BMP) and the ABG are within 2 points of each other.[9] If these results are not within 2 points of 1 another, the results are uninterpretable.[9]

Step 2: Determine the Primary Disorder

The next step is to look at the pH and determine if there is acidemia (pH <7.4) or alkalemia (pH >7.4). After this is determined, the $Paco_2$ should be looked at. If the pH and $Paco_2$ are going in the same direction, the primary disorder is metabolic.[6] If the pH and $Paco_2$ are going in the opposite direction, the primary disorder is respiratory.[6]

Step 3: If the Primary Disorder Is Respiratory, Determine if It Is Acute or Chronic

An acute respiratory disorder is classified as a condition that has been present less than 24 hours, whereas a chronic respiratory disorder is a condition that has been present more than 3 days.[9] To determine if the respiratory disorders are acute or chronic, the calculations provided in step 3 of **Table 2** should be used.

Step 4: Calculate the Anion Gap

Calculation of the anion gap (AG) is essential to analyzing acid-base disorders correctly. To maintain electroneutrality of the extracellular fluid, the sum of the concentration of the positively charged cations and negatively charged anions must be equal.[8] An AG can be calculated to measure if there is an imbalance in the positive- and negative-charged substances in the blood. The AG is calculated by using the following formula and the results of the BMP[6,8,9]:

$$AG = [Na^+] - ([CL^-] + [HCO_3^-])$$

A normal AG is around 12 mEq/L.[6,8,9] It is important to note that it is necessary to correct the AG if the patient has a low albumin level. For every 1 g/dL drop in albumin less than 4.0 g/dL, there is a corresponding 2.5 mEq/L decrease in the AG.[9] If an AG is present, the patient has an AG metabolic acidosis, and the differential diagnosis is outlined in **Table 3** by using the mnemonic GOLD MARK.[9,11] In other stepwise approaches to

Table 2
Stepwise approach to arterial blood gas interpretation

Step	Description
1. Gather all the necessary data	ABG and BMP
2. Determine the primary disorder	Look at the pH: Does the pH indicate acidemia or alkalemia? Look at the $Paco_2$: • Are the pH and $Paco_2$ going in the same direction? (Metabolic) • Are the pH and $Paco_2$ going in opposite directions? (Respiratory)
3. If the primary disorder is respiratory, determine if it is acute or chronic	Respiratory acidosis: • Acute: For every 1-point increase in $Paco_2$ >40, there should be a pH decrease of 0.008. • Chronic: For every 1-point increase in $Paco_2$ >40, there should be a pH decrease of 0.003. Respiratory alkalosis: • Acute: For every 1-point decrease in $Paco_2$ <40, there should be a pH increase of 0.008. • Chronic: For every 1-point decrease in $Paco_2$ <40, there should be a pH increase of 0.003.

4. Calculate the AG	$AG = [Na^+] - ([Cl^-] + [HCO_3])$
	Correct the AG for albumin. For every 1 g/dL drop in albumin <4.0 g/dL, there is a corresponding 2.5 mEq/L decrease in the AG.
	If AG is >12, an AG metabolic acidosis is present, so it is necessary to:
	• Calculate the delta gap:
	  ○ delta gap = Calculated AG – 12
	• Calculate the corrected or potential HCO_3
	  ○ Corrected or potential HCO_3 = delta gap + measured HCO_3
	If corrected HCO_3 is >26, a metabolic alkalosis is also present.
	If corrected HCO_3 is <22, a non-AG metabolic acidosis is also present.

5. Apply formulas to determine if compensation is appropriate or if secondary (mixed) disorder is present	Metabolic disorders: Calculate the expected $Paco_2$ ($\Delta PaCO_2$ + 40)
	• Metabolic acidosis: $\Delta PaCO_2$ = 1.2 × change in HCO_3
	  ○ The $Paco_2$ will decrease 1 unit for every 1.2 unit decrease in HCO_3
	• Metabolic alkalosis: $\Delta PaCO_2$ = 0.7 × change in HCO_3
	  ○ The $Paco_2$ will increase 1 unit for every 0.7 unit increase in HCO_3
	• If actual $Paco_2$ > expected, concomitant respiratory acidosis.
	• If actual $Paco_2$ < expected, concomitant respiratory alkalosis.
	Respiratory disorders: Calculate the expected HCO_3
	(HCO_3 = ΔHCO_3 + 24)
	• Respiratory acidosis:
	  ○ Acute: ΔHCO_3 = 1 mEq/L increase for every 10 mm Hg increase in $Paco_2$
	  ○ Chronic: ΔHCO_3 = 3 mEq/L increase for every 10 mm Hg increase in $Paco_2$
	• Respiratory alkalosis:
	  ○ Acute: ΔHCO_3 = 2 mEq/L decrease for every 10-mm Hg decrease in $Paco_2$
	  ○ Chronic: ΔHCO_3 = 4 mEq/L decrease for every 10 mm Hg decrease in $Paco_2$
	• If actual HCO_3 < expected HCO_3, concomitant metabolic acidosis.
	• If actual HCO_3 > expected HCO_3, concomitant metabolic alkalosis.

6. Look at the Pao_2 and SaO_2 for signs of hypoxemia	Mild hypoxemia: SaO_2 90%–94% and Pao_2 60–79 mm Hg Moderate hypoxemia: SaO_2 75%–89% and Pao_2 40–59 mm Hg Severe hypoxemia: SaO_2 <75% and Pao_2 <40 mm Hg

Abbreviations: Cl^-, chlorine ion; Na^+, sodium ion; pH, acidity.
Data from Refs.[4,6,8–10]

Table 3
The differential diagnosis for acid-base disorders

AG Metabolic Acidosis	Non-Gap Metabolic Acidosis	Acute Respiratory Acidosis	Metabolic Alkalosis	Respiratory Alkalosis
GOLD MARK	**ACCRUED**	**CHOMPP**	**CLEVER PD**	**CHAMPS**
Glycols (ethylene and propylene)	Acid load	CNS depression	Contraction	CNS disease
Oxoproline	Carbonic anhydrase inhibitors	Hemothorax (pneumothorax)	Licorice	Hypoxia
L-Lactate	Chronic kidney disease (renal failure)	Obstruction (airway)	Endo Conn, Cushing, & Bartter	Anxiety
D-Lactate	Renal tubular acidosis	Myopathy	Vomiting	Mechanical ventilators
Methanol	Uretero-enterostomy	Pneumonia	Excess alkali	Progesterone: pregnancy and liver disease
Aspirin	Expansion (volume)	Pulmonary edema	Refeeding alkalosis	Salicylates and sepsis
Renal failure	Diarrhea	Anything that causes hypoventilation of chronic respiratory acidosis (COPD and restrictive lung disease)	Posthypercapnia	Anything that causes hyperventilation
Ketoacidosis (EtOH, starvation, DKA)			Diuretics	

Abbreviations: CNS, central nervous system; DKA, diabetic ketoacidosis; EtOH, ethanol.
From DeWaay D, Gordon J. The ABC's of ABG: teaching arterial blood gases to adult learners. MedEdPORTAL. 2011;7(9038). https://doi.org/10.15766/mep_2374-8265.9038; with permission.

ABG interpretation,[6] the AG calculation is completed as the first step of ABG analysis to narrow the differential diagnosis for the acid-base disorder earlier in the diagnostic process. Whether it is the first or last step of the ABG analysis, it is imperative always to calculate the AG, because it may expose a hidden metabolic disturbance.

If the AG is normal, the last step in the ABG analysis process is complete. If the AG is increased, the next step is to calculate the delta gap and then the corrected or potential HCO_3 using the following formulas[6,9]:

- Delta gap = Calculated AG − 12
- Corrected or potential HCO_3 = delta gap + measured HCO_3

For example, if the AG is 18 and the measured HCO_3 is 9, the delta gap is 6 (18 − 12) and the corrected HCO_3 would be 15 (6 + 9). Use the following guidelines to interpret these results:

- If the corrected HCO_3 is greater than 26, a metabolic alkalosis is present in addition to the AG metabolic acidosis.
- If the corrected HCO_3 is less than 22, non-AG metabolic acidosis is present in addition to the AG metabolic acidosis.[9]

Step 5: Apply Formulas to Determine if Compensation Is Appropriate. If Not, a Concomitant Disorder Coexists (ie, a Mixed Acid-Base Disorder)

In this step, application of the various formulas for each of the 6 acid-base disorders will result in determining if compensation for the acidemia or alkalemia is appropriate or if a concomitant acid-base disorder coexists.[9] For example, if an ABG yields a pH 7.28 and an HCO_3 of 13 (indicating a primary metabolic acidosis), use of the formula in **Table 2** (step 5) for metabolic acidosis indicates the following[9]:

- The HCO_3 decreased by 11, so the $Paco_2$ should go down by 13.2 (1.2 × 11 = 13.2).
- The expected $Paco_2$ is 26.8 (40 − 13.2 = 26.8).
- The actual $Paco_2$ is 27, so there is no concomitant disorder.

For primary respiratory disorders, the formulas found in step 5 of **Table 2** can be applied to determine if the HCO_3 compensation is appropriate or if a secondary acid-base disorder is present. As a general rule, compensation for chronic respiratory acidosis/alkalosis will be higher than in acute respiratory disorders because there has been ample time for the kidneys to respond to the pH imbalance. For instance, in acute respiratory acidosis, as the $Paco_2$ increases, the HCO_3 will start to go up, but only a small amount (approximately 1 mEq/L for every 10 mm Hg increase in $Paco_2$), because the renal compensation is just beginning and is not complete.[8] However, in chronic respiratory acidosis, there has been enough time for the kidneys to fully adjust the HCO_3 to its new steady state value, so the compensation formula predicts a greater HCO_3 value than in acute compensation (HCO_3 increases by 3 mEq/L for every 10 mm Hg increase in $Paco_2$).[9] Similarly, for respiratory alkalosis, the formulas for calculating the predicted HCO_3 account for the difference between appropriate compensation for acute and chronic respiratory disorders. For both acute and chronic respiratory disorders (acidosis and alkalemia), if the actual HCO_3 differs significantly from the expected, then a coexisting metabolic disorder is present.[9]

Step 6: Look at the Pao_2 and Sao_2 for Signs of Hypoxemia

The last step in the stepwise approach to ABG interpretation is to look at the Pao_2 and SaO_2 for signs of hypoxemia.[10] When there are low levels of oxygen in the blood (as evidenced by lower than normal Pao_2 and Sao_2), the patient has hypoxemia. When the pH of the blood is abnormal, oxyhemoglobin dissociation is impaired and less oxygen gets to the tissues, resulting in hypoxemia.[5] Hypoxemia causes a shift to anaerobic respiration, which can lead to lactic acid buildup, increasing the severity of acidemia.[5] Step 6 of **Table 2** outlines a classification system for hypoxemia and can be used in ABG interpretation of these values.

When the Pao_2 and Sao_2 values are abnormal, their results can be used to calculate more accurate assessments of oxygenation[12]:

- The alveolar-arterial gradient
- Ratio of Pao_2/fraction of inspired oxygenation
- Oxygen delivery

More thorough descriptions or calculations of these more exact measurements of oxygenation, pulmonary gas exchange, and ventilation are beyond the scope of this review; however, PAs wishing to learn more about these indices of oxygenation and their utility in patient care should refer to the references provided in this article.

CONDITIONS CAUSING ACID-BASE IMBALANCE: CASE-BASED APPLICATIONS

The differential diagnosis for the 6 types of acid-base disorders (with helpful mnemonics for ease of recall) is presented in **Table 3**. This tool will be instrumental in helping to establish the diagnosis of an acid-base disorder after interpreting an ABG. With this information on the differential diagnosis and the steps in the ABG analysis process, it is time to apply the approach to 3 case presentations.[9]

Case 1

A 40-year-old woman with a past medical history significant for cirrhosis of the liver secondary to alcoholism has a BMP HCO_3 of 17. An ABG showed a pH 7.46; $Paco_2$, 20; Pao_2, 80; HCO_3, 16; and Sao_2, 95% on room air. The AG was 10, and albumin, 4.0.

The pH, in this case, shows an alkalemia (pH >7.4). The pH and the $Paco_2$ are going in opposite directions (pH is up; $Paco_2$ is down), so the primary disorder is respiratory alkalosis. Applying the formulas provided in step 3 of **Table 2** shows that the patient has a chronic respiratory alkalosis because the pH will increase by 0.06 ($0.003 \times 20 = 0.06$), thereby yielding a pH 7.46. There is no AG, and the albumin is normal, so no adjustments need to be made. For step 5, the formula for respiratory alkalosis is applied (change in HCO_3 = 4 mEq/L decrease for every 10 mm Hg decrease in $Paco_2$). The $Paco_2$ is down by 20, so it is expected that the HCO_3 would go down by 8. Expected HCO_3 is 16 ($24 - 8 = 16$), so there is no concomitant metabolic disorder. The Pao_2 and Sao_2 are both normal, so there is no concern for hypoxemia.

The final interpretation is chronic respiratory alkalosis.

Case 2

A 75-year-old man with a history of systolic congestive heart failure and chronic kidney disease presents with a 3-day history of increasing dyspnea, 4.5 kg weight gain, lower-extremity edema, and orthopnea. His creatinine is at his baseline. An ABG showed a pH 7.25; $Paco_2$, 46; Pao_2, 78; HCO_3, 20; and Sao_2, 94% on 2 L oxygen. The AG was 10, and albumin, 4.0.

The pH shows an acidemia. The pH and $Paco_2$ are going in opposite directions (pH is down; $Paco_2$ is up), so the primary disorder is respiratory acidosis. Formulas from step 3 are then used to determine if the respiratory acidosis is acute or chronic. The $Paco_2$ has increased by 6; if this is chronic respiratory acidosis, the pH will decrease by 0.02 and would be 7.38 ($0.003 \times 6 = 0.018$; $7.4 - 0.02 = 7.38$). If this is an acute respiratory acidosis, the pH will decrease by 0.05 and would be 7.35 ($0.008 \times 6 = 0.048$; $7.4 - 0.05 = 7.35$). Because this value is closer to the actual pH, this is acute respiratory acidosis. There is no AG, and an albumin correction is not necessary. Based on the formula provided in step 5, the $Paco_2$ is up by 6, so the HCO_3 should go up by 0.6 (1-mEq/L increase for every 10 mm Hg the $Paco_2$ goes up). Expected HCO_3 is 24.6 ($24 + 0.6 = 24.6$), and actual HCO_3 is 20. Because the actual HCO_3 is less than the expected, the patient has a concomitant metabolic acidosis. The Pao_2 and SaO_2 are slightly lower than normal, indicating the patient has (at a minimum) mild hypoxemia.

The final interpretation is respiratory acidosis with concomitant non-AG metabolic acidosis.

Case 3

A 22-year-old man with a history of bipolar disorder was brought by ambulance to the emergency department after ingesting a bottle of aspirin in a suicide attempt. An ABG showed a pH 7.38; $Paco_2$, 23; Pao_2, 84; HCO_3, 16; and SaO_2, 98% on room air. The AG was 18, and albumin, 4.0.

The patient has an acidemia (pH <7.4), and the pH and $Paco_2$ are going in the same direction (both decreased), so the primary disorder is metabolic acidosis. The AG is elevated. The albumin is normal, so no correction is needed. The delta gap is 6 ($18 - 12 = 6$). The corrected HCO_3 is 22 ($6 + 16 = 22$), so there is no concurrent metabolic disturbance. Based on the formula provided in step 5 of **Table 2**, the $Paco_2$ will decrease 1 unit for every 1.2 units the HCO_3 decreases, so the expected $Paco_2$ is 30.4 ($1.2 \times [24 - 16] = 9.6$; $40 - 9.6 = 30.4$). The actual $Paco_2$ (23) is less than the expected $Paco_2$ (30), so there is concomitant respiratory alkalosis. The Pao_2 and SaO_2 are within normal limits, indicating there is no hypoxemia.

The final interpretation is AG metabolic acidosis with concomitant respiratory alkalosis.

SUMMARY

ABG analysis is an essential aspect of diagnosing and managing a patient's oxygenation status and acid-base balance; however, its usefulness is highly dependent on correctly interpreting the results. PAs must learn and master this skill. A thorough understanding of acid-base physiology is essential to the ABG interpretation process, and as with other skills, such as electrocardiogram or x-ray interpretation, a systematic approach and regular practice with application of that approach are necessary to gain competence and confidence in this skill.

REFERENCES

1. Sood P, Paul G, Puri S. Interpretation of arterial blood gas. Indian J Crit Care Med 2010;14(2):57–64.
2. Theodore AC. Arterial blood gases. In: Manaker S, Finlay G, editors. UpToDate. Waltham (MA): UpToDate; 2018.
3. Cameron P. Textbook of adult emergency medicine. 4th edition. Edinburgh (Scotland): Churchill Livingstone; 2015.
4. Singh V, Khatana S, Gupta P. Blood gas analysis for bedside diagnosis. Natl J Maxillofac Surg 2013;4(2):136–41.

5. Larkin BG, Zimmanck RJ. Interpreting arterial blood gases successfully. AORN J 2015;102(4):343–54.

6. MedCram. Medical acid base balance, disorders & ABGs explained clearly 2017. YouTube. https://www.medcram.com/. Accessed July 19, 2018.

7. Barnette L, Kautz DD. Creative ways to teach arterial blood gas interpretation. Dimens Crit Care Nurs 2013;32(2):84–7.

8. Preston RA. Acid-base, fluids, and electrolytes made ridiculously simple. 3rd edition. Miami (FL): MedMaster, Inc; 2018.

9. DeWaay D, Gordon J. The ABC's of ABG: teaching arterial blood gases to adult learners, vol. 7. MedEdPORTAL; 2011. p. 9038.

10. Burns GP. Arterial blood gases made easy. Clin Med (Lond) 2014;14(1):66–8.

11. Mehta AN, Emmett JB, Emmett M. GOLD MARK: an anion gap mnemonic for the 21st century. Lancet 2008;372(9642):892.

12. Marino PL. The ICU book. 3rd edition. Philadelphia: Lippincott Williams & Wilkins; 2014.

Renal Function Testing

Patricia G. Martin, BS-MT (ASCP), MBA, PA-C

KEYWORDS

- Urinalysis • Estimated glomerular filtration rate (eGFR) • Renal markers
- Chronic renal failure • Acute kidney injury

KEY POINTS

- Although current guidelines recommend against routine screening of individuals without risk factors, new World Health Organization (WHO) recommendations include routine point-of-care screening for all individuals.
- Proper diagnosis, staging, and management of chronic kidney disease (CKD) or acute kidney injury (AKI) incorporate good clinical judgment and proper interpretation of laboratory data.
- The preferred initial studies for evaluating renal function are urinalysis and serum creatinine with estimated glomerular filtration rate (eGFR). These do not accurately reflect onset of AKI, however.
- Newer calculations and novel biomarkers show better efficacy in establishing accurate eGFR in both CKD and AKI.
- Urine protein, urine electrolyte analysis, imaging, and renal biopsy are helpful to confirm underlying renal pathologic condition.

INTRODUCTION

The kidneys control fluid volume, plasma osmolality, acid-base, and electrolyte balance and remove metabolic wastes and toxins via the nephron. These processes can be measured by laboratory means to establish kidney health, diagnose renal injury, stage the degree of insufficiency, and monitor therapy. Knowing the condition of the kidney also allows for appropriate drug dosing to reduce risk of acute kidney injury (AKI).

The indications for screening and frequency of testing are somewhat controversial. Current guidelines recommend that only those patients at significant risk for developing renal failure be routinely screened.[1–4] In May 2018, the World Health Organization (WHO) Strategic Advisory Group on In Vitro Diagnostics published their first "Essential Diagnostics List," which recommends routine screening by urine dipstick plus blood urea nitrogen (BUN) and serum creatinine (SCr) levels for all individuals at the lowest 2 tiers of care (primary care clinic and hospital).[5]

Disclosure Statement: The author have no relationship, financial or otherwise with any commercial organization referenced in this article.
Physician Assistant Program, Marietta College, Marietta, OH, USA
E-mail address: pamarietta65@gmail.com

Physician Assist Clin 4 (2019) 561–578
https://doi.org/10.1016/j.cpha.2019.02.007
2405-7991/19/© 2019 Elsevier Inc. All rights reserved.

	Definitions
Chronic kidney disease (CKD)	Progressive decline of GFR over a period of >3 mo, usually associated with albuminuria
Acute kidney injury (AKI)	Increase in serum creatinine $\geq$0.3 mg/dL above the previously established baseline within 48 h or presumed to occur within the previous 7 d Or when urine output drops $\leq$3 mL/kg over a 6-h period
Renal failure	Advanced end-stage chronic kidney disease (ESRD)
Glomerular filtration rate (GFR)	The sum-total of plasma filtrate from all functional nephrons in 1 min. Normal is considered 120 mL/min or >60 mL/min/1.73 m^2 (m^2 = body surface area)
Specific gravity (SG)	The measure of the concentration of solutes in urine expressed as a ratio of urine density to pure water density
Sterile pyuria	White blood cells in numbers >5/hpf, without bacteriuria and negative urine culture

LET THE HISTORY AND PHYSICAL GUIDE YOU

Kidney disease may be symptomatic or asymptomatic, chronic or acute, and may influence or stress the function of any organ of the body. With more than 25 major causes of chronic kidney disease (CKD) and innumerable systemic, genetic, or iatrogenic factors contributing to AKI, when and what to test must be informed by the individual's risk factors (**Table 1**). For example, hospitalized patients have risk factors for AKI that warrant ongoing monitoring 6 months after discharge, and pediatric patients with history of anemia, neonatal hypertension, or other conditions that may affect renal perfusion should be monitored for progressive renal disease.

WHICH LABORATORY TESTS AND WHEN

The preferred first choices for routine point-of-care (POC) screening are urinalysis (UA) and basic or comprehensive metabolic panel (BMP/CMP), including BUN and SCr, with estimated glomerular filtration rate (eGFR, [in mL/min/1.73 m^2]). At a minimum, this basic screening should be ordered for all pregnant women at first visit and regularly during gestation, all hospitalized patients at admission and preoperatively, and any patient with a chief complaint of abdominal pain, back pain, dysuria, hematuria, polyuria, or significant risk of developing CKD.[1] Other reasons the clinician may wish to screen for renal disease include

- To rule out/in changes in renal function
- To Monitor renal function in confirmed CKD
- To reveal underlying causes of abnormal UA results
- To Document the degree of functional loss
- Before initiating or changing medications

URINALYSIS

The most cost-effective and readily available laboratory evaluation is the UA. This test assesses the kidney's work over the previous 24 hours and can suggest renal tubular or parenchymal damage. It cannot determine the degree of functional loss. The best specimen is a freshly voided, clean catch, midstream urine. Occasionally, a first morning collection or 24-hour collection is warranted.

Table 1
Some common indications for renal function screening

History/Comorbidity	Renal Implications	Recommended Screening
Diabetes	CKD	UA, CBC, BMP, HgA$_{1c}$
Hypertension (HTN): Neonatal HTN, chronic uncontrolled HTN	CKD in adults AKI in infants	UA, CBC, BMP
Cardiovascular disease Sepsis, shock, CV surgery	CKD, AKI, acute on chronic	UA, CBC, BMP, Troponin, ECG
Smoking	CKD	UA, CBC, BMP
Infection: E coli HIV, HBV, HCV, poststreptococcal	CKD, AKI, hemolytic uremic syndrome	UA, CBC w/platelet, BMP, Shiga toxin, complement, viral screen and titer, IgA, ASO titers
Anemia: Sickle cell, leukemia	AKI with progression to CKD	UA, CBC, BMP
Heavy metal exposure rhabdomyolysis	AKI	UA, CBC, BMP, lead level, others prn
Autoimmune disorders	CKD, AKI, acute on chronic	UA, CBC, BMP, ANA, ANCA (PR3-ANCA and MPO-ANCA)
Recurrent acute events: nephrolithiasis, pyelonephritis	AKI with progression to CKD	UA, CBC, BMP, imaging
Iatrogenic: Recent hospitalization Contrast dye & medication	AKI, AKI with progression to CKD	UA, CBC, BMP daily during admission & 6 mo after discharge

Abbreviations: ANA, antinuclear antibody panel; ANCA, antineutrophil cytoplasmic antibodies; BMP, basic metabolic panel; CBC, complete blood count with platelets; CV, cardiovascular; ECG, electrocardiogram; HBV & HCV, hepatitis B and C virus; HgA$_{1c}$, hemoglobin A1C; HIV, human immunodeficiency virus; MPO-ANCA, myloperoxidase antibodies; PR3-ANCA, Proteinase 3 antibodies; UA, urinalysis.

Gross Appearance

Generally, observation of the specimen's color, consistency, and odor is a poor indicator of disease, but red or brown urine suggests glomerular disease, urinary tract infection (UTI), or renal calculi.

Dipstick Analysis

A urine dipstick (**Fig. 1**) is an easily executed test for a variety of biochemical markers. Results are read by comparison with a color chart or automated analyzer. Careful compliance with the manufacturer's package insert will provide the most accurate result.

- Urine pH: Acid-base hemostasis takes place in the renal tubules by excretion of hydrogen ions and selective excretion and reabsorption of bicarbonate. Normal urine pH may fluctuate between 4.5 and 8.5. In the setting of normal renal function, abnormal urine pH implies a systemic acidemia or alkalosis that may be influenced by diet[6] or respiratory illness. However, normal to elevated urine pH in the setting of acidemia suggests chronic renal failure or renal tubular acidosis (RTA).
- Specific Gravity: Urine specific gravity (SG) is an indicator of the kidney's ability to concentrate urine, prevent excessive fluid loss, and balance electrolytes. Normal adult urine SG ranges from 1.010 to 1.030 (in neonates as low as

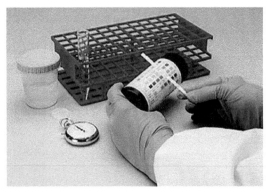

Fig. 1. Example of dipstick UA. (*From* Kathleen Pagana D, Pagana JT, Pike-MacDonald SA. Mosby's Canadian manual of diagnostic and laboratory tests, Second Canadian edition, Philadelphia: Elsevier, 2019, Figure 11.1.)

1.003). Increased SG is almost always associated with prerenal causes (dehydration, heart failure, renal stenosis, and so forth), but may suggest abnormal levels of glucose, proteins, or insoluble elements. Decreased SG accompanies renal failure, pyelonephritis, acute tubular necrosis (ATN), interstitial nephritis, and other nonrenal causes. When SG is significantly abnormal by dipstick, confirmation by refractometry or direct osmometry provides greater accuracy and is less influenced by large undissolved particles.[7]

- Protein: Any amount of protein in urine is abnormal and an important indicator of renal disease. Current international guidelines include urine protein as a parameter for staging CKD.[1] The dipstick test for protein has several limitations and interfering conditions (**Table 2**). Most significantly:
  - It is designed to detect albumin not light chain proteins (may nonselectively detect high concentrations of mucoproteins and globulins).
  - It is sensitive to albumin at levels greater than 15 to 30 mg/dL and does not reliably detect moderate increase (microalbuminuria) as seen in diabetics. A separate microalbumin test strip is available.
  - It is semiquantitative (1+, 2+, 3+), and sensitivity depends on urine concentration (SG).
- Heme: The test pad for blood detects the presence of heme in any form (intact red blood cells [RBC], free hemoglobin, or myoglobin). False results are detailed in **Table 2**. All heme-positive specimens should be confirmed by microscopic examination and should trigger further investigation for a source.
- Nitrite: Infection anywhere along the urinary tract may be detected by either positive nitrite or positive leukocyte esterase (LE), or both. Nitrites are produced when urea is metabolized by urease-producing gram-negative bacteria, which include the most common causes of UTI (*Escherichia coli* and *Klebsiella pneumoniae*).[8] Other common UTI organisms (Pseudomonas, Streptococcus, Staphylococcus, and Enterococcus) do not produce nitrate reductase and are not detected by nitrite alone.
- Leukocyte Esterase: Leukocytes infiltrating the area will produce large amounts of esterase enzymes, which are detected by the LE strip. Confusion may arise when the nitrite and LE tests are not coincidentally positive. Microscopic UA (see "*Microscopic Urine Analysis*") is helpful. Exclusive reliance on UA has resulted in overtreatment of sterile pyuria in hospitalized patients.[9,10] Culture and

Table 2
Sources of false results on dipstick

Dipstick Test	Falsely Elevated/Positive	Falsely Decreased/Negative
pH	UTI from ammonia-producing bacteria Vegetarian diet	UTI by urease-producing bacteria Diets high in meat or cranberry juice
SG	High levels of large molecules (glucose, proteins, radiocontrast, buffering agents) Dehydration or other prerenal causes	AKI Polyuria, polydipsia Urine pH >6.5
Protein	Vaginal discharge or semen Hematuria Highly concentrated urine	Highly dilute urine
Heme (blood)	Menses, semen Hemolytic anemia, coagulopathies Trauma Microvascular disease Rhabdomyolysis Starvation Malignant hyperthermia Glycogen storage disease	High intake of ascorbic acid (vitamin C)
LE	Contaminated specimen	Glucosuria Proteinuria Some common antibiotics
Nitrite	None	Reduced urine retention Nonnitrite reductase-producing UTI (proteus, pseudomonas, enterococci)

sensitivity should follow all positive screens or when infection is suspected, but dipstick is negative. Symptoms suggesting pyelonephritis also warrant imaging (see "*Imaging*").

- Glucose: Glucosuria is an indicator of hyperglycemia at levels that overwhelm the proximal tubule's ability to reabsorb glucose. Some congenital, genetic, and acquired renal conditions (ie, RTA, Fanconi syndrome) may result in glucosuria when plasma glucose levels are normal. The sensitivity of the test strip can be as low as 75 mg/dL glucose. Patients who consistently test trace to 100 mg/dL glucose should be evaluated further for renal causes.

Microscopic Urine Analysis

Urine microscopic examination is part of a full UA done in the laboratory. Urine sediment is concentrated by centrifugation and examined under the microscope. Cellular components are quantified, and casts, crystals, bacteria, and fungi are characterized.

- Cells: Positive dipstick findings are confirmed by observing RBCs, white blood cells (WBCs), bacteria or fungal elements, and epithelial cells (**Table 3**). The significance of cellular findings includes the following:
  - Transitional or tubular epithelial cells are concerning for renal disease. Large, broad squamous epithelial cells originate from the bladder and urethra.[11]
  - Significant WBCs with bacterial or fungal elements, in symptomatic patients, is adequate evidence to initiate empiric treatment of UTI pending culture.
  - Sterile pyuria (see "*Definitions*") suggests interstitial nephritis, nephrolithiasis, or atypical infections (tuberculosis, chlamydia, and similar).[10]

Table 3
Significance of cellular components found in urine

Cell Type	Abnormal Threshold	Cause	Adjunctive Testing
RBC	≥2 RBCs/hpf		
	Benign	Vaginal contamination, menstrual vs postcoital bleeding	Vaginal examination
	Transient	Strenuous exercise, cystitis	Repeat UA, culture
	Persistent	Malignancy, glomerular disease, renal calculi	US, biopsy, + crystals
	Dysmorphic RBCs	Glomerular disease, prerenal RBC destruction	Proteinuria on dipstick, CBC, serology
WBC	≥2–5 WBCs/hpf		
	With bacteria/fungi	UTI, pyelonephritis	Gram stain, reflex culture, imaging
	No bacterial/fungi	Interstitial nephritis, renal TB, nephrolithiasis	AFB stain/culture, imaging, biopsy
Epithelial cells	>15–20 cells/hpf (large, broad, flat SEC)	Generally contamination	
	>15 cells/hpf (transitional or renal tubule)	ATN, exposure to nephrotoxin, transplant rejection	Imaging or biopsy

Abbreviations: AFB, acid-fast bacilli; hpf, high-power field; SEC, squamous epithelial cells; TB, tuberculosis; US, renal ultrasound.

- o Special staining for urine eosinophils is no longer recommended to confirm acute interstitial nephritis.[12]
- Crystals: Crystals can be a risk factor for development of renal calculi or diagnostic for known kidney stones. Crystal morphology is specific to their composition (**Table 4**). Conditions that favor the formation of crystals include pH and urine concentration (ie, dehydration or stasis).
- Casts: Cylindrical molds of the renal tubules mainly consisting of Tamm-Horsfall mucoprotein are called casts. Casts are significant for the cells trapped within the matrix:
  - o Clear hyaline casts are acellular and may be present in highly concentrated urine, in the setting of urine stasis, or in low urine pH of a normal individual.
  - o Cellular casts suggest renal disease based on the type of cells found (**Table 5**).[13]
  - o Broad casts are typically formed in the large distal tubules of individuals in late-stage CKD.
- Lipiduria: Fat droplets (seen as "Maltese Crosses" under polarized light) may be free in urine, in sloughed tubular epithelial cells, or in fatty casts. Small numbers of free fat droplets are not concerning, but large numbers of droplets, fatty casts, or coexisting tubular epithelial cells are strong evidence for glomerular disease, polycystic kidney disease, interstitial nephritis (acute and chronic), or prerenal azotemia.

ASSESSING FUNCTIONAL RENAL TISSUE
Blood Urea Nitrogen, Serum Creatinine

As the kidney fails, nitrogenous waste in the form of urea and by-products of metabolism (principally creatinine) increases progressively. The measure of BUN and SCr

Table 4
Common urinary crystals associated with renal disease

Crystal	Composition	Contributing Factors	Associated Pathologic Condition
	Uric acid	Acid pH	Acute uric acid nephropathy, chronic urate nephropathy, uric acid stones
	Calcium oxalate	Non-pH dependent, hypercalciuria	Renal calculi: Calcium stones
	Calcium phosphate	Alkaline pH, hypercalciuria	Less common cause of calcium stones
	Cystine	Cystinuria	Genetic disorder
	Struvite (magnesium ammonium phosphate)	Elevated ammonia Alkaline pH	Staghorn calculi, recurrent UTI (urease-producing bacteria)
	Calcium carbonate	Alkaline pH, low urine citrate, normal serum bicarbonate, ± hypercalciuria	Distal RTA

Photos reprinted from Beňovská Miroslava, and Ondřej Wiewiorka, Faculty of Medicine, Masaryk University. Microscopic analysis of urine. https://is.muni.cz/do/rect/el/estud/lf/js15/mikroskop/web/index_en.html, with permission; and *From* Lenka Michalková, Servistech, Interactive and Multimedia Learning Support Center for Learning Innovation and Effective Learning.

reflects recent renal function (within 3 hours) and can be used to stage functional renal tissue. Because several extrarenal factors affect these markers, significant clinical judgment is necessary when interpreting the data (**Table 6**). The BUN-to-creatinine ratio can be examined to quickly narrow the differential diagnosis to prerenal, intrarenal, or postrenal conditions (**Fig. 2**). However, this does not stage the degree of functional lost.

Table 5
Common urinary casts associated with renal disease

Casts	Composition	Contributing Factors	Associated Pathologic Condition
	Clear hyaline cast (Tamm-Horsfall mucoprotein without cells)	Acid pH Stasis Concentrated urine	Dehydration, urinary tract obstruction, diet
	Erythrocyte cast	Nephritic syndromes Vasculitis	Acute nephritis, IgA nephropathy, lupus nephritis, pyelonephritis
	WBC cast	Tubulointerstitial disease	Acute pyelonephritis, acute interstitial nephritis, lupus nephritis, acute papillary necrosis
	Renal epithelial cell cast	Viremia Nephrotoxin exposure	ATN
	Granular cast	Intense physical activities or cold exposure, urinary stasis, degraded cellular casts	Any tubulointerstitial disease associated with cellular cast formation
	Waxy cast	Stasis and nephron obstruction	Severe CKD Amyloidosis
	Fatty cast	Elevated triglycerides Uncontrolled diabetes	Diabetic nephropathy, nephritic syndromes
	Bacterial cast	Recurrent UTI, sepsis	Chronic pyelonephritis, renal abscess

Photos reprinted from Beňovská, Miroslava and Ondřej Wiewiorka, Faculty of Medicine, Masaryk University. Microscopic Analysis of Urine. https://is.muni.cz/do/rect/el/estud/lf/js15/mikroskop/web/index_en.html, with permission; and *From* Lenka Michalková, Servistech, Interactive and Multimedia Learning Support Center for Learning Innovation and Effective Learning.

Table 6
Extrarenal causes for abnormal blood urea nitrogen and serum creatinine

	BUN	Serum Creatinine
Elevated	High-protein diet	Shock
	Gastrointestinal bleeding	Dehydration
	Urinary outlet obstruction	Congestive heart failure
	Congestive heart failure	Atherosclerosis
	Recent heart attack	Diabetes
	Dehydration	Rhabdomyolysis
	Shock	High-protein intake (less than for BUN)
	Severe burns	
	Steroids	
	Fever	
	Rhabdomyolysis	
Decreased	Severe liver disease	Low muscle mass
	Malnutrition	Low protein diet
	Overhydration	

The best indicator of functional nephron loss is the glomerular filtration rate (GFR). Direct measurement of GFR (the gold standard) requires administration of a soluble, freely filtered exogenous marker (usually inulin or iothalamate) with collection and testing of a 24-hour urine specimen. This method is cumbersome and impractical for most POC applications.

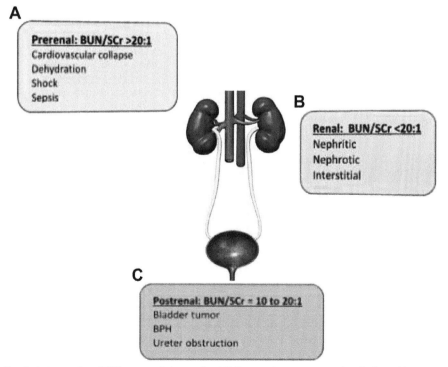

A

Prerenal: BUN/SCr >20:1
Cardiovascular collapse
Dehydration
Shock
Sepsis

B

Renal: BUN/SCr <20:1
Nephritic
Nephrotic
Interstitial

C

Postrenal: BUN/SCr = 10 to 20:1
Bladder tumor
BPH
Ureter obstruction

Fig. 2. Interpreting BUN-to-creatinine ratio. (*A*) Prerenal causes occurring before filtration; (*B*) renal causes occurring due to kidney disease; (*C*) postrenal causes occurring after filtration.

Traditionally, creatinine-based methods have been used to indirectly estimate the GFR (**Table 7**); however, creatinine has considerable variation among "normal" populations owing to variations in muscle mass, gender, age, race, body surface area, and nutritional status. Since Cockcroft-Gault formula was first proposed (1976),[14] attempts have been made to normalize and standardize this estimate. Two alternative equations now widely accepted as standard for eGFR in adults are the following:

- Modification of Diet in Renal Disease (MDRD-eGFR)[15,16]
- Chronic Kidney Disease Epidemiology Collaboration (CKD-EPI)[17]

Current international guidelines recommend using CKD-EPI.[1,18] However, only 4% of US laboratories use this formula.[19] MDRD-eGFR (with correction for African American race) predominates. Evidence suggests that CKD-EPI is more accurate at

Table 7
Common equations for estimating glomerular filtration rate

Equation Name	Equation	Marker	Comments
Creatinine clearance	$GFR = \dfrac{[UrCr \times V]}{SCr}$	SCr	Cumbersome 24-h urine collection unreliable
Cockcroft-Gault	$eGFR = \dfrac{(140 - age) \times weight}{72 \times SCr}$ (multiply weight by 0.85 if ♀)	SCr	Accuracy varies w/obesity, ethnicity Not standardized to current methods Overestimates GFR 10% to 40%[13]
[a]MDRD-eGFR	$eGFR = 175 \times SCr^{-1.154} \times Age^{-0.203} \times 0.742\ (if\ ♀)$ Result must be corrected for race	SCr	Most used by laboratories in United States Accuracy varies by ethnicity Most accurate at normal to near-normal GFR
[b]CKD-EPI	$eGFR = 141 \times min\ (SCr/κ, 1)^{α} \times max\ (SCr/κ, 1)^{-1.209} \times 0.993^{Age} \times [1.018\ (if\ ♀)] \times [1.159\ (if\ Black)]$	SCr	More precise at lower range of GFR May affect staging of moderate to severe CRD
[b]SCy-C MDRD or CKD-EPI	Substitute SCy-C level for SCr	SCy-C	Requires overnight fast Best to confirm questionable eGFR, ESRD, and transplant candidates
[b]Schwartz	$eGFR = 41.3 \times (height/SCr)$	SCr	Recommended by KDIGO 2017 Standardized to pediatric population
MDRD or CKD-EPI [b]Combined analysis	See on-line calculators	SCr + SCy-C	Considered best calculation for end-stage and renal transplant patients

Abbreviations: age in years; height in meters; weight in kg; max, maximum of $S_{Cr}/κ$ or 1; min, minimum of $S_{Cr}/κ$ or 1; SCy-C, serum cystatin-C; the constant κ in the Schwartz formula refers to age adjusted muscle mass; UrCr, urine creatinine; V, volume; α, −0.329 (women) or −0.411 (men); κ, 0.7 (women) or 0.9 (men).

[a] MDRD-eGFR most commonly reported by US laboratories.
[b] Highest recommendation. Online calculators and mobile applications are available.

predicting CKD in patients at or near normal GFR, whereas both are comparable when used to stage more advanced CKD.[19–21]

Because body mass in children is not equivalent to adults, the Schwartz equation[22] uses the child's height and is recommended in pediatric populations.[1,23] This calculation varies based on the creatinine assay method used (Jaffe vs enzymatic method). Only the enzymatic method is recommended.[1,22] In children less than 2 years old, normal eGFR is less than 60 mL/min/1.73 m.

The use of creatinine-based procedures assumes that creatinine is produced at a stable rate and freely filtered, but creatinine is also secreted by the renal tubules. It has been shown that this may result in as much as 40% overestimation of GFR.[24] Additional sources of error in creatinine-based assays are detailed in the Kidney Disease: Improving Global Outcomes (KDIGO) guidelines (**Table 8**). Most notably, in the setting of AKI, unstable creatinine negates the efficacy of these formula (see "*Evaluating Acute Kidney Injury*"). Therefore, these methods are only used to diagnose and stage CKD.

Serum Cystatin-C

Recent efforts have focused on identifying other biomarkers that are produced at constant levels and freely filtered by the glomerulus.[25] The most studied of these compounds is cystatin-C (SCy-C), a metabolite produced at a constant rate by all

Table 8
Sources of error in glomerular filtration rate estimating using creatinine

Source of Error	Example
Nonsteady state	• AKI
Non-GFR determinants of SCr that differ from study populations in which equations were developed Factors affecting creatinine generation	• Race/ethnicity other than US and European black and white • Extremes of muscle mass, Extremes of body size • Diet and nutritional status ○ High-protein diet, ingestion of cooked meat ○ Creatine supplements • Muscle wasting diseases
Factors affecting tubular secretion of creatinine	• Decrease by drug-induced inhibition ○ Trimethoprim ○ Cimetidine ○ Fenofibrate
Factors affecting extrarenal elimination of creatinine	• Dialysis • Decrease by inhibition of gut creatininase by antibiotics • Increased by large volume losses of extracellular fluid
Higher GFR	• Higher biological variability in non-GFR determinants relative to GFR ○ Higher measurement error in SCr and GFR
Interference with creatinine assay	• Spectral interferences (eg, bilirubin, some drugs) • Chemical interferences (eg, glucose, ketones, bilirubin, some drugs) • Inaccurate 24-h urine collection

Reprinted with permission from International Society of Nephrology. KDIGO clinical practice guideline for evaluation and management of chronic renal failure. 2012.

nucleated cells, freely filtered, and nearly completely reabsorbed by the renal tubule. Although widely used internationally, it is not standardized for eGFR in the United States but is available as an add-on laboratory test (on-line calculators exist for $eGFR_{SCy-C}$ calculation at POC). Evidence shows that SCy-C may be better at predicting AKI but not better than MDMR or CKD-EPI at staging CKD.[20,26] Therefore, SCy-C should be reserved for use in prognosticating AKI (see "Evaluating Acute Kidney Injury"), when creatinine-based estimates are confusing or unexpected, when staging end-stage renal failure (ESRF), or when evaluating patients for renal transplant.[20,27] Combining both SCr and SCy-C in 1 equation has also shown increased precision.[27]

Evaluating Acute Kidney Injury

Rapid decline in renal function is the hallmark of AKI, yet eGFR lags symptoms. Currently, in critical care settings, fluid intake and urine output (I&Os), urine albumin, SCr with eGFR, and electrolytes are monitored continuously for early onset AKI.[28] These laboratory studies are neither preemptive nor standard procedure for general hospital or outpatient populations. In at least 1 study, as many as 6.7% of the general hospital population (not admitted to critical care units) developed AKI.[29]

The use of combined SCr/SCy-C[25,27,30] or novel biomarkers, like tissue inhibitor of metalloproteinase-2 and insulin-like growth factor binding protein-7 (NephroCheck, Astute Medical, Inc),[31] has been reported to be effective predictors of AKI in postoperative and critical care populations, but have not been studied in the general population.

In settings outside critical care, clinical judgment must be used to anticipate risks for AKI. If one relies exclusively on eGFR, the opportunity to intervene early and preserve renal tissue is missed. Additional testing provides data on cause and severity of injury:

- For hospitalized patients, daily I&Os and BMP or CMP (for SCr, eGFR, BUN, and electrolytes) will provide early data, allowing for aggressive fluid management and removal or dose modification of offending drugs.
- In outpatient settings, all patients should be screened after discharge or after exposure using UA with microscopy and eGFR by SCr.
- Urine electrolytes, especially fractional excretion of sodium (FENa), will help to differentiate the cause of injury (see "Urine Electrolytes").
- CBC, serologies, imaging, biopsy, and others are helpful when the cause of injury is uncertain.

LABORATORY TESTS WHICH DIFFERENTIATE RENAL DISEASE

Given the broad differential for renal disease, it is necessary to exercise good clinical judgment when deciding which panel of tests to order. Components of the patient history and physical examination and previous laboratory testing, imaging, or renal biopsy will aid in focusing the investigation and limiting cost (**Table 9**).

Urine Protein

The presence, character, and quantity of protein in urine are important indicators for renal disease. Clinical albuminuria of greater than 30 mg/dL suggests glomerulonephritis, renal tubular disease, infection (ie, pyelonephritis, cystitis), preeclampsia of pregnancy, or amyloidosis.

Proteinuria on dipstick should be rechecked and quantified, and a urine albumin-to-creatinine ratio (ACR) or protein-to-creatinine ratio (PCR) reported.[1,32] The amount and type of protein are important differentiating features in determining glomerular

Table 9
Additional testing for differentiation and cause of renal disease

Laboratory Test	History and Physical Findings	Underlying Pathologic Condition
Serum uric acid	History of gout or renal stones Uremic symptoms	Renal calculi Heavy metal poisoning
Acid-fast culture	Exposure history, + skin test, + CXR	Renal TB
HIV screen and titer	Fever of unknown origin Recurrent infections Exposure history IV drug abuse	HIV-AIDS nephritis
Hepatitis B & C	Exposure history IV drug abuse Elevated liver enzymes	Viral nephritis
Heavy metal levels Other toxicology	History of exposure Lead ingestion and poisoning	AKI Hyperuricemia Proximal tubular dysfunction RTA
Coagulation studies	Unexplained bruising Postprocedure bleeding history	Minimal change disease, Henoch- Schönlein purpura Disseminated intravascular coagulation
Serologic testing: ANAs ASO titer RF Complement	History of joint pain, fevers, recurrent infections Recent streptococcal infection Lung hemorrhage Nephritis w/o hemorrhage Lower extremity purpura Granuloma	Acute tubular nephritis IgA nephritis Pauci-Immune glomerulonephritis Goodpasture Anti-GBM nephritis Cryoglobulin glomerulonephritis
Erythropoietin	Anemia of chronic disease	Late-stage CKD and ESRD
25-hydroxyvitamin D, alkaline phosphate, serum phosphate, parathyroid hormone	Renal bone disease	Late-stage CKD and ESRD
Biopsies immunoassay	Any signs or symptoms of: Nephritic syndrome Nephrotic syndrome CKD AKI Autoimmune disorders	Nephritic & nephrotic disease Nonspecific changes CKD Sclerotic lesions Mesangial cell proliferation Amyloid Congo Red stain Wegner granulomatosis Wright stain for eosinophilia Autoimmune nephropathy Specific immunofluorescent stains

Abbreviations: ASO, antistreptolysin-O; CXR, chest x-ray; IV, intravenous; RF, rheumatoid factor; w/o, without.

from nonglomerular disease. Suspected false negative dipstick results should also undergo sulfosalicylic acid testing and protein electrophoresis to identify light-chain proteins.

Although the gold standard for quantitative protein analysis is a 24-hour total urine protein, a simpler method uses a random spot ACR or PCR. A ratio of 0.2 is normal and

Fractional excretion of sodium is the ratio of sodium clearance to creatinine clearance.

$$FENa = \frac{Urine\ Na \times Plasma\ Cr}{Plasma\ Na \times Urine\ Cr} \times 100$$

Where:

FENa <1% Prerenal, glomerulonephritis, obstruction
FENa >2% Acute Tubular Necrosis
FENa 1–2% Equivocal

Fig. 3. FENa. Cr, creatinine; Na, sodium.

correlates with a 24-hour excretion of less than 200 mg of protein[33] (>150 mg/d is abnormal). One to 2 g per day is usually significant for glomerular disease, whereas less than 1 g/d is more likely to occur in the tubules. Urine protein of greater than 3.5 g/d is consistent with a diagnosis of nephrotic syndrome.

The source of proteinuria can be characterized as glomerular, tubular, functional, postrenal, or overflow, whereby

- *Glomerular proteinuria* is albumin, positive by dipstick, and suggests nephrotic or nephritic syndromes
- *Tubular proteinuria* is low-molecular-weight protein, not detected by dipstick, normally reabsorbed in the proximal tubules, and suggests nephritic syndromes when less than 2 g/d
- *Functional proteinuria* is transient, less than 1 g/d, and typically occurs in young healthy adults, confirmed by split samples (AM and PM).
- *Postrenal proteinuria* is associated with infection, positive for nitrites and/or LE, numerous WBCs and bacteria, and is confirmed by culture
- *Overflow proteinuria* results from high plasma concentration of abnormal low-molecular-weight proteins (Bence-Jones proteins, myoglobin, paraproteins, and hemoglobin), not detected by dipstick, that overwhelm the reabsorption capacity of the proximal tubule.

Urine Electrolytes

Fractional excretion of electrolytes and other substances (urea and uric acid) may be used to differentiate tubular insufficiency. FENa (**Fig. 3**) is most commonly used in the setting of AKI.[34] Because plasma concentration of sodium depends on intake, FENa only has efficacy for differentiating prerenal loss of perfusion from ATN in the setting of known AKI. It is not a reliable measure in neonates or small children.[35] Fractional excretion of other substances (potassium, chloride, urea, and uric acid) has greater utility in evaluating extrarenal pathologic condition.[36]

IMAGING

Multiple imaging modalities may be considered based on the suspected pathologic condition (**Table 10**). Imaging assists in staging CKD and diagnosing interstitial renal disease, polycystic kidney disease, and congenital or genetic defects of the kidney.

Convenience, breadth of utility, the ability to avoid contrast media, and the noninvasive nature of ultrasound (US) or Doppler US make it the first choice for imaging the kidney. The kidney's size, echogenicity, and position can be measured, revealing masses (solid tumor vs cyst vs abscess), small size, and cortical thickening of CKD

Table 10
Renal imaging procedures and their applications

Imaging Modality	Application	Comments
Renal US	Differentiating renal mass Detecting hydronephrosis Proximal obstructing stone Renal parenchymal disease Pyelonephritis	Preferred first choice for evaluation
Doppler US	Renal vascular flow obstruction Stenosis Thrombosis	Less sensitive than CTA Normal resistive index <0.7
CT	Nonobstructing stones Evaluating and staging masses Localization of obstructions Congenital malformation	Low-dose noncontrast CT is gold standard for renal calculi
MRI	Characterization of tumor or cyst Genetic or congenital disorders	Used when use of contrast media is contraindicated
Plain abdominal radiograph	Rarely used Safe in pregnant & pediatric patients	Low sensitivity and specificity May detect some radiopaque stones
Intravenous pyelography	Detecting stones and obstructions of urinary tract	Uses iodinated contrast media Process slower than CT
Renal arteriography/ venography (CTA or MRA)	Evaluation of renal vasculature Thrombosis Renal artery stenosis	Mapping blood supply to tumor before surgery
Radionuclide studies	Vesicoureteral reflux in children Assess renal perfusion	Lacks specificity for renal filtration studies

and renal parenchymal disease (ie, renal calcinosis in RTA). US can often diagnose hydronephrosis due to obstruction, masses, strictures, or stones in the renal pelvis or proximal ureter (sensitivity is diminished in the distal ureter due to overlying bowel). The addition of Doppler flow studies provides information on the perfusion of the kidney and facilitates early intervention in the setting of renal ischemia or infarct due to renal stenosis, thrombosis, or other vascular defects.

Computed tomography (CT), CT angiography (CTA), MRI, and MRI with angiography (MRA) constitute the next level of radiographic investigation providing complementary information on intrarenal and renovascular pathologic condition. Drawbacks to these procedures include increased exposure to radiation with CT and the use of contrast media. The FDA now recommends that SCr with eGFR be rechecked in patients with known eGFR less than 60 mL/min/1.73 m^2 48 hours after exposure to gadolinium (MRI, MRA) to prognose nephrogenic systemic fibrosis.[37]

BIOPSY

Renal biopsy is undertaken when laboratory data are equivocal, when transplant rejection is suspected, or when there is systemic disease with renal involvement. The most common procedure is US- or CT-guided percutaneous needle aspirate. Laparoscopic, transjugular, or open approaches are also possible. Renal biopsy is not done for low-grade or transient proteinuria or intermittent hematuria. Relative contraindications include bleeding disorders or congenital malformation of the kidney. The tissue is examined by plain light, immunofluorescent, and electron microscopy (see **Table 9**).

MONITORING CONFIRMED RENAL DISEASE

Once renal disease is confirmed, continuous or intermittent monitoring is recommended to follow progression or recovery of function. Baselines for eGFR, urine albumin, serum calcium, phosphate, parathyroid hormone, and vitamin D should be established for all patients at risk for CKD. Individuals with known CKD should be monitored annually for albuminuria and eGFR.[1] All patients with recent hospitalizations should be evaluated at 6 months after discharge, and those with history of AKI should be evaluated at 3 months.[28] Current guidelines recommend against routine screening of individuals without risk factors, but the WHO now recommends eGFR and urine albumin annually.[5] Any evaluation beyond these minimum recommendations should be based on clinical judgment, patient risk, and changes in medication.

SUMMARY

Good clinical judgment and proper interpretation of laboratory data are critical to diagnosis and management of renal disease. Controversy exists with respect to the most efficacious method of estimating GFR, whether to routinely test asymptomatic individuals without risks, and how often to test those with risk factors. In the United States, the MDRD is most widely used to calculate and report eGFR. Internationally, CKD-EPI and CKD-EPI$_{SCy-C}$ are standard. SCy-C levels with online or mobile calculators may be used at POC when necessary. It is important to remember that eGFR is only accurate in stable conditions (ie, normal function or CKD). Other biomarkers should be used when prognosing AKI.

REFERENCES

1. Official Journal of the International Society of Nephrology, Kidney Disease: Improving Global Outcomes (KDIGO) CKD Work Group. KDIGO 2012 Clinical practice guideline for the evaluation and management of chronic kidney disease. Kidney Int Suppl 2013;3(1):4.
2. Moyer VA, on behalf of the U.S. Preventive Services Task Force. Screening for chronic kidney disease: U.S. preventive services task force recommendation statement. Ann Intern Med 2012;157:567–70.
3. Qaseem A, Hopkins RH, Sweet DE, et al. For the Clinical Guidelines Committee of the American College of Physicians. Screening, Monitoring, and Treatment of Stage 1 to 3 Chronic Kidney Disease: A Clinical Practice Guideline From the American College of Physicians. Ann Intern Med 2013;159:835–47.
4. Baumgarten M, Gehr T. Chronic kidney disease: detection and evaluation. Am Fam Physician 2011;84(10):1138–48.
5. World Health Organization. Model list of essential in vitro diagnostics. Geneva (Switzerland): WHO Press; 2018. p. 35. Available at: https://www.ghdonline.org/uploads/EDL_ExecutiveSummary_15may.pdf. Accessed May, 2018.
6. Welch AA, Mulligan A, Bingham SA, et al. Urine pH is an indicator of dietary acid-base load, fruit and vegetables and meat intakes: results from the European Prospective Investigation into Cancer and Nutrition (EPIC)-Norfolk population study. Br J Nutr 2008;99(6):1335–43.
7. De Buys Roessingh AS, Drukker A, Guignard JP. Dipstick measurements of urine specific gravity are unreliable. Arch Dis Child 2001;85(2):155–7.
8. Behzadi P, Behzadi E, Yazdanbod H, et al. A survey on urinary tract infections associated with the three most common uropathogenic bacteria. Maedica

(Buchar) 2010;5(2):111–5. Available at: http://www.ncbi.nlm.nih.gov/pubmed/21977133%5Cnhttp://www.pubmedcentral.nih.gov/articlerender.fcgi?artid=PMC3150015. Accessed May, 2018.

9. Keller SC, Feldman L, Smith J, et al. The use of clinical decision support in reducing diagnosis of and treatment of asymptomatic bacteriuria. J Hosp Med 2018;13(6):392–5. Available at: https://www.journalofhospitalmedicine.com/jhospmed/article/152882/hospital-medicine/use-clinical-decision-support-reducing-diagnosis-and. Accessed July, 2018.

10. Turpen HC. Frequent urinary tract infection. Physician Assist Clin 2018;3(1):55–67.

11. Butterworth STG. Cells in the urine. Br Med J 1968;4(5629):517.

12. Ruffing KA, Hoppes P, Blend D, et al. Eosinophils in urine revisited. Pediatr Nephrol 1995;9(2):198.

13. Ringsrud KM. Casts in the urine sediment. Lab Med 2001;32(4):191–3.

14. Cockcroft DW, Gault MH. Prediction of creatinine clearance from serum creatinine. Nephron 1976;16:31–41. Available at: https://www.ncbi.nlm.nih.gov/pubmed/1244564. Accessed May, 2018.

15. Levey AS, Bosch JP, Lewis J, et al. A more accurate method to estimate glomerular filtration rate from serum creatinine: a new prediction equation. Modification of Diet in Renal Disease Study Group. Ann Intern Med 1999;130(6):461–70. Available at: https://doi.org/10.7326/0003-4819-130-6-199903160-00002. Accessed May, 2018.

16. Hallan S, Åsberg A, Lindberg M, et al. Validation of the modification of diet in renal disease formula for estimating GFR with special emphasis on calibration of the serum creatinine assay. Am J Kidney Dis 2004;44(1):84–93.

17. Levey AS, Stevens LA, Schmid CH, et al. A new equation to estimate glomerular filtration rate. Ann Intern Med 2009;150(9):604–12.

18. National Institute for Health and Care Excellence (NICE). General guideline 182: chronic kidney disease in adults: assessment and management 2014. Available at: https://www.nice.org.uk/guidance/cg182/chapter/1-Recommendations#investigations-for-chronic-kidney-disease-2. Accessed June, 2018.

19. Matsushita K, Mahmoodi BK, Woodward M, et al. Comparison of risk prediction using the CKD-EPI equation and the MDRD study equation for estimated glomerular filtration rate. JAMA 2012;307(18):1941–51.

20. Inker LA, Levey AS, Coresh J. Estimated glomerular filtration rate from a panel of filtration markers—hope for increased accuracy beyond measured glomerular filtration rate? Adv Chronic Kidney Dis 2018;25(1):93–104.

21. Delanaye P, Pottel H, Botev R. Con: should we abandon the use of the MDRD equation in favour of the CKD-EPI equation? Nephrol Dial Transplant 2013;28(6):1396–403. Available at: https://doi.org/10.1093/ndt/gft006. Accessed May, 2018.

22. Abraham AG, Schwartz GJ, Furth S, et al. Longitudinal formulas to estimate GFR in children with CKD. Clin J Am Soc Nephrol 2009;4(11):1724–30.

23. Selistre L, Rabilloud M, Cochat P, et al. Comparison of the Schwartz and CKD-EPI equations for estimating glomerular filtration rate in children, adolescents, and adults: a retrospective cross-sectional study. PLoS Med 2016;13(3):e1001979.

24. Peralta CA, Katz R, Sarnak MJ, et al. Cystatin C identifies chronic kidney disease patients at higher risk for complications. J Am Soc Nephrol 2011;22(1):147–55.

25. Wu I, Parikh CR. Screening for kidney diseases: older measures versus novel biomarkers. Clin J Am Soc Nephrol 2008;3(6):1895–901.

26. Murty MSN, Sharma U, Pandey V, et al. Serum cystatin C as a marker of renal function in detection of early acute kidney injury. Indian J Nephrol 2013;23(3):180.

27. Zhang W, Zhang T, Ding D, et al. Use of both serum cystatin C and creatinine as diagnostic criteria for contrast-induced acute kidney injury and its clinical implications. J Am Heart Assoc 2017;6(1):e004747.
28. Moore PK, Hsu RK, Liu KD. Management of acute kidney injury: core curriculum 2018. Am J Kidney Dis 2018;72(1):136–48.
29. Kashani K, Shao M, Li G, et al. No increase in the incidence of acute kidney injury in a population-based annual temporal trends epidemiology study. Kidney Int 2017;92(3).
30. Nice. The NGAL Test for early diagnosis of acute kidney injury. p. 1–35. Available at: http://publications.nice.org.uk/the-ngal-test-for-early-diagnosis-of-acute-kidney-injury-mib3/technology-overview. Accessed June, 2018.
31. Lowes R. FDA oks Nephrocheck to assess risk for acute kidney injury. MedScape Med News 2018. Available at: https://www.medscape.com/viewarticle/831212. Accessed June, 2018.
32. Kellum JA, Lameire N, Aspelin P, et al. KDIGO clinical practice guideline for acute kidney injury. Kidney Int Suppl 2012;2(1):1–138.
33. Hasanato RM. Diagnostic efficacy of random albumin creatinine ratio for detection of micro and macro-albuminuria in type 2 diabetes mellitus. Saudi Med J 2016;37(3):268–73.
34. Schreuder MF, Bökenkamp A, Van Wijk JAE. Interpretation of the fractional excretion of sodium in the absence of acute kidney injury: a cross-sectional study. Nephron 2017;136(3):221–5.
35. Ellis EN, Arnold WC. Use of urinary indexes in renal failure in the newborn. Am J Dis Child 1982;136(7):615–7. Available at: https://doi.org/10.1001/archpedi.1982.03970430047013. Accessed June, 2018.
36. Schrier RW. Diagnostic value of urinary sodium, chloride, urea, and flow. J Am Soc Nephrol 2011;22(9):1610–3.
37. US Food and Drug Administration. FDA drug safety communication: new warnings for using gadolinium-based contrast agents in patients with kidney dysfunction 2010. Available at: https://www.fda.gov/Drugs/DrugSafety/ucm223966.htm. Accessed June, 2018.

Provider-Performed Microscopy Procedures

Annamarie Faust Streilein, MT(ASCP), MHS, PA-C[a,b,*]

KEYWORDS

- Provider-performed microscopy • Point-of-care testing • Wet mount • KOH testing
- Pinworm examination • Fern test • Microscopic urinalysis • Nasal smear

KEY POINTS

- Rapid on-site clinical laboratory testing can improve quality of patient care and increase patient satisfaction.
- Microscopic testing of patient specimens that may degrade during transport to the centralized laboratory may be performed at the point of care to increase test result quality and patient convenience.
- Clinicians, including physician assistants, may perform provider-performed microscopy (PPM) procedures if all relevant Clinical Laboratory Improvement Amendment (CLIA) requirements are met.
- There are 9 CLIA-approved PPM procedures.

 Video content accompanies this article at http://www.physicianassistant. theclinics.com.

INTRODUCTION
Clinical Scenario

A woman comes to your clinic with a complaint of 3-day history of yellow vaginal discharge with an unpleasant odor. After you take her history, perform a focused physical examination, and collect a specimen of discharge from the vaginal wall, you order a wet mount and then learn that your laboratory technologist is in a meeting for the next 2 hours. You believe it is likely you will be able to make a definitive diagnosis as soon as you get the wet mount result. In the interest of time, should you perform the wet mount yourself?

Disclosure Statement: The author has no commercial or financial conflicts of interest to disclose.
[a] Duke Physician Assistant Program, Department of Family Medicine and Community Health, Duke University Medical Center, DUMC 104780, Durham, NC 27710, USA; [b] Alamance County Health Department, Burlington, NC, USA
* Duke Physician Assistant Program, Department of Family Medicine and Community Health, Duke University Medical Center, DUMC 104780, Durham, NC 27710, USA.
E-mail address: annamarie.streilein@duke.edu

Physician Assist Clin 4 (2019) 579–589
https://doi.org/10.1016/j.cpha.2019.02.004
2405-7991/19/© 2019 Elsevier Inc. All rights reserved.

Answer

Maybe, but it depends on several factors. See the clinical scenario update at the end of this article.

CONTENT
Background

Clinicians, including physicians, physician assistants (PAs), nurse practitioners, nurse midwives, and dentists, use point-of-care tests (POCTs) in the medical care of their patients.[1] As these tests are performed outside a centralized laboratory, at or near the patient, involve minimal instrumentation, and have a quick turnaround time, the use of such tests can provide rapid diagnostic information, enhance the quality of care and patient satisfaction, and reduce cost.[1–3] In some medical settings, these tests can actually be performed by the clinician.[4] Medical settings in which clinicians may be more likely to perform POCT include rural clinics, urgent care clinics, primary care practices, emergency departments, health departments, sexually transmitted disease clinics, community health centers, or some specialty practices.

US medical sites where POCTs are performed are required to meet federal regulatory standards of the Clinical Laboratory Improvement Amendment (CLIA) of 1988.[5] All clinical laboratory testing performed on humans in the United States, except clinical trials and basic research, is required to meet these standards.[5] On request by the test manufacturer, the US Food and Drug Administration (FDA) assigns each in vitro diagnostic test a category according to its degree of complexity, and categorizes each test as waived, moderate complexity, or high complexity.[6] These 3 categories are based on an assessment of the requirements to perform each test, and graded in 7 areas, including the level of scientific and technical knowledge; training and experience; reagent safety and reliability; complexity of specimen preparation or test operation; calibration, quality control, and proficiency testing materials; test system troubleshooting and equipment maintenance; and interpretation and judgment.[6] The CLIA test categorization is based on the FDA determination of test complexity. Per the code of federal regulations (CFR) 493.15c,[7] all testing sites are required to have a CLIA certificate issued by the Centers for Medicare and Medicaid Services (CMS) before testing patient specimens.

Waived Tests

As the CLIA category of least complex diagnostic tests, waived tests are agreed to be simple to perform, unlikely to provide incorrect information, and unlikely to cause harm if misperformed. All tests that are waived under CFR 493.15c or approved for over-the-counter or home use fall into this category.[7] There are currently 132 tests that have been granted waived status by CLIA.[8] Clinicians, including PAs, can perform these tests if the clinical practice laboratory has a CLIA certificate of waiver, and follows all the associated requirements. These requirements include paying the biannual certificate renewal fee, notifying the state agency within 30 days of any change in laboratory ownership, name, address or director, and allowing on-site inspections by CMS.[7]

Moderate-Complexity Tests

Laboratories may qualify for a CLIA certificate of moderate complexity if it limits testing to waived tests in addition to 1 or more examinations or tests that qualify as moderate complexity, including provider-performed microscopy (PPM) procedures.[9] PPM procedures are a specific subcategory of moderate-complexity tests. PPM is a testing modality that requires the use of a microscope and is performed by physicians or nonphysician practitioners during the patient's visit.[4] Microscopic observation of clinical specimens at the point of care allows for rapid detection of pathologic findings. Diagnostic quality can be improved from testing or examination of fresh specimens in which formed elements are less likely to degrade. Clinicians, including PAs, can perform PPM procedures as part of the patient visit if their clinic has a CLIA certificate of accreditation for PPM, and in addition follows all the PPM procedure-associated requirements. Application for this CLIA certificate for PPM procedures requires completion of the CMS-116 form.[10] Unlike the large number in the waived test category, there are only 9 PPM procedures[9] (**Box 1**).

This article focuses on a practical review of the PPM procedure subset of moderate-complexity tests.

High-Complexity Tests

High-complexity tests require more complicated equipment, training, procedure, and supplies, or longer turnaround time than waived tests or PPM procedures. Clinical laboratories in which high-complexity tests are performed are required to hold a CLIA certificate of accreditation specifically for high-complexity tests. CLIA does not support performance of high-complexity tests by clinicians.

Provider-Performed Microscopy Procedures

Each of the 9 PPM procedures is reviewed in this section. Refer to **Table 1** for an overview of PPM specimens, potential findings, procedure, and diagnostic utility.

Wet Mount

The wet mount, also called wet prep, involves microscopic visualization of cells and organisms in a specimen collected and suspended in 0.5 to 1.0 mL 0.9% saline for identification, morphology and motility. Vaginal wet mount specimens should be collected from the walls of the vagina with a wooden or plastic scraper or a cotton swab and immediately placed in a tube containing room temperature saline. If assessed, the vaginal pH should be determined and documented before adding the specimen to the saline tube.[2,11] A vaginal pH greater than 4.5 is associated with

---

Box 1

Clinical Laboratory Improvement Amendment–approved provider-performed microscopy procedures

Wet mount (all direct wet mount) preparation for the presence or absence of bacteria, fungi, parasites, and human cellular elements

Potassium hydroxide (KOH) preparation

Pinworm examination

Fern test

Postcoital direct, qualitative examination of vaginal or cervical mucus

Urine sediment examination

Nasal smear for granulocytes

Fecal leukocyte examination

Qualitative semen analysis (limited to the presence or absence of sperm and detection of motility)

Table 1
Summary of provider-performed microscopy (PPM) procedures

PPM Procedure	Specimen	Procedure Summary	Findings	Diagnostic Utility
Wet mount	Vaginal secretions	Microscopic visualization of cells and organisms in saline suspension for identification, morphology, and motility; pH of vaginal specimens.	Bacteria, *Trichomonas vaginalis*, clue cells, yeast, white blood cells, red blood cells, squamous epithelial cells, artifacts	Evaluation of vaginitis.
Potassium hydroxide (KOH) preparation	Vaginal secretions, skin scraping, hair, nails	Addition of 10% KOH solution digests obscuring keratin, epithelial cells, and white blood cells for improved microscopic visualization of yeast and fungi. Amine odor in KOH-exposed vaginal specimen indicates overgrowth of anaerobic bacteria.	Hyphae, pseudohyphae, spores; amine odor (vaginal specimen)	Evaluation of suspected superficial fungal infections (vagina, skin, hair, or nails).
Pinworm examination	Superficial perianal	Microscopic identification of pinworm eggs in a superficial specimen from perianal skin folds collected onto sticky surface.	*Enterobius vermicularis* eggs	Evaluation of *pruritis ani*; *E vermicularis* diagnosis.
Fern test	Vaginal fluid	Leaked amniotic fluid air-dried on microscope slide is examined.	Crystallized amniotic fluid in fern pattern	Evaluation of suspected preterm prelabor rupture of fetal membrane; fertility monitoring.
Postcoital direct, qualitative examination of vaginal or cervical mucus	Postovulation, postintercourse cervical mucus	Specimen collected from cervical os via syringe is assessed for mucus volume, color, clarity, and viscosity; sperm number and motility.	Vaginal mucus color, viscosity, and tenacity; sperm presence and motility	Fertility evaluation.

Urine sediment examination	Urine	Formed elements in urinary sediment concentrated via centrifugation are identified and enumerated microscopically.	Cells, casts, crystals, microorganisms, artifacts	Support diagnosis of multiple renal and urinary tract disorders.
Nasal smear for granulocytes	Nasal discharge	Nasal discharge specimen is applied to slide, air-dried, stained, and examined microscopically for increased eosinophils.	Eosinophils in nasal secretions	Rhinitis evaluation: support diagnosis of allergic etiology.
Fecal leukocyte Examination	Feces	Fecal specimen is applied to slide, air-dried, stained, and examined microscopically for leukocytes.	Leukocytes in fecal smear	Bacterial infection such as shigellosis, or differentiation between inflammatory and noninflammatory diarrheas.
Qualitative semen analysis	Semen	Fresh semen specimen is applied to slide and examined microscopically for presence of sperm. If present, % forward motility is determined.	Presence or absence of sperm; sperm motility	Infertility evaluation, vasectomy effectiveness, evaluation of semen for artificial insemination.

bacterial vaginosis or trichomoniasis.[11] Preparations should be examined within 60 minutes of collection, and ideally within 10 to 15 minutes,[2] to avoid degradation of formed elements or death of easily identifiable motile trichomonads.[12] The wet mount may be done in conjunction with the potassium hydroxide (KOH) preparation. Wet mount results can confirm diagnoses of trichomoniasis (**Fig. 1**), bacterial vaginosis (**Fig. 2**), yeast vaginitis (**Fig. 3**), mucopurulent cervicitis, and support diagnoses of chlamydia, gonorrhea, or genital herpes. Diagnostic yield is highest in vaginal wet mount specimens collected in the absence of recent intravaginal medications or douching.[2]

Potassium Hydroxide Preparation

The KOH preparation is used to evaluate suspected superficial fungal infections. In the KOH preparation, a 10% KOH solution is added to a specimen on a slide to digest obscuring keratin, epithelial cells and white blood cells (WBCs) in samples of vaginal secretions, skin scrapings, hair, or nails so yeast and fungi can be identified microscopically. Additional detection of an amine odor in a KOH-exposed vaginal specimen (also known as the "whiff test"[2]) indicates overgrowth of anaerobic bacteria.

Pinworm Examination

The pinworm examination, or pinworm paddle test, involves microscopic identification of pinworm eggs in a superficial specimen from the perianal skin folds collected onto a sticky surface and placed on a microscope slide (**Fig. 4**). It is most commonly performed on patients, often children, presenting with perianal itching. Obtaining the specimen at night or early in the morning before toileting or bathing, provides the greatest diagnostic yield. The eggs have a characteristic bean shape, with flattening on one side, and their visualization is diagnostic of an *Enterobius vermicularis* infection.

Fern Test

The fern test detects amniotic fluid leakage or elevated estrogen secretion in vaginal specimens. It is most commonly used to confirm a diagnosis of preterm prelabor rupture of fetal membranes. The fern test is usually done after determining the pH of the vaginal specimen with Nitrazine paper, which helps differentiate among normal vaginal fluid, urine, and amniotic fluid. For the fern test, a specimen of fluid from the posterior vaginal fornix is swabbed onto a glass slide and allowed to dry for 10 minutes, then examined microscopically. Dried amniotic fluid arborizes on the microscope slide, crystallizing into a fern pattern (**Fig. 5**). The presence of this characteristic fern pattern is a positive test.

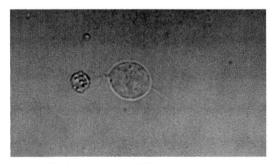

Fig. 1. Vaginal wet prep: *Trichomonas* and WBCs. Unstained saline wet mount, original magnification 400×. (*Courtesy of* Jane McDaniel, MS, MLS, SC)

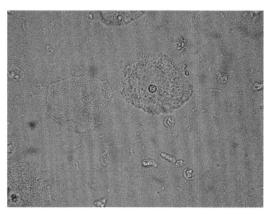

Fig. 2. Vaginal wet prep: normal squamous epithelial cell and clue cell. Unstained saline wet mount, original magnification 400×. (*Courtesy of* Jane McDaniel, MS, MLS, SC)

Postcoital Direct Qualitative Examination

The postcoital direct qualitative examination of vaginal or cervical mucus test, or postcoital test, is performed on a postovulation, postintercourse cervical mucus specimen removed from the cervical os via syringe. The mucus volume is measured and color and clarity are observed. Viscosity is assessed by measuring a strand of mucus drawn from the droplet on the slide. The number and motility of sperm in mucus is assessed microscopically. The goal of this test is to assess cervical mucus receptivity and the ability of sperm to penetrate mucus as one component of fertility evaluation. This test is now felt to have limited clinical utility and is not generally recommended by fertility specialists.[13]

Urine Sediment Examination

Urine sediment examination, also called microscopic urinalysis or urine microscopy, is an important optional component of complete urinalysis. It is primarily used if there are positive findings on chemical ("dipstick") urinalysis, which also may be performed by the provider via dipstick, tablet reagent, or waived automated urinalysis instrument.[14] In urine sediment examination, 10 to 12 mL of a well-mixed, room

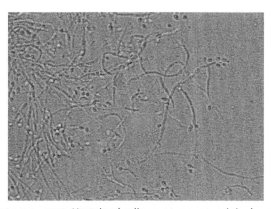

Fig. 3. Vaginal wet prep: yeast. Unstained saline wet mount, original magnification 400×. (*Courtesy of* Jane McDaniel, MS, MLS, SC)

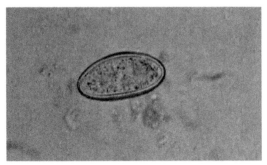

Fig. 4. Scotch tape prep: pinworm egg. Unstained saline wet mount, original magnification 400×. (*Courtesy of* Jane McDaniel, MS, MLS, SC)

temperature fresh urine specimen is centrifuged for 5 minutes at 704 x *g*, which concentrates the formed elements. The supernatant is decanted and discarded, and the remaining urinary sediment pellet is resuspended with or without a drop of stain. A small drop of the mixed sediment is placed on a microscope slide and a coverslip is applied (commercially prepared slides with built-in cover slips are available.) Clinically significant formed elements, including cells (WBCs, red blood cells, and epithelial cells), microorganisms (bacteria, fungi, and motile trichomonads), casts, and crystals are identified with the light microscope. Lipid-rich elements and some crystals are best visualized with polarizing light. Casts are enumerated at ×100 total magnification and all other elements are enumerated at ×400. Urine sediment examination is extremely helpful in the evaluation of suspected urinary tract disorders and renal diseases.

Nasal Smear for Granulocytes

The nasal smear for granulocytes is sometimes referred to as nasal cytology. In this test, a specimen of nasal discharge is collected onto a cotton swab and applied to a slide, air-dried, stained, and examined microscopically for increased eosinophils. Evaluation of other cells is not included in this PPM procedure. Although relatively insensitive and nonspecific, the presence of nasal eosinophilia is suggestive of an allergic rather than infectious etiology for increased nasal secretions. The test also may be used to assess response to anti-inflammatory therapy via noting reduction in nasal eosinophilia.

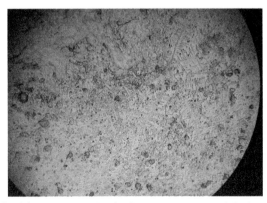

Fig. 5. Amniotic fluid ferning. Unstained saline wet mount, original magnification 400×. (*Courtesy of* Jane McDaniel, MS, MLS, SC)

Fecal Leukocyte Examination

In fecal leukocyte examination (sometimes called stool microscopy), a fecal specimen is applied to a slide, air-dried, stained, and examined microscopically for leukocytes. Fecal leukocytes may be assessed with or without fecal occult blood testing and if positive, may be helpful supporting a diagnosis of inflammatory diarrhea, such as shigellosis.[15] Stool microscopy might also include identification of parasitic organisms such as helminths (cysts, eggs, larvae) and protozoa, but note that this component of stool microcopy is not an approved PPM procedure.

Qualitative Semen Analysis

In qualitative semen analysis, a fresh semen specimen is applied to a slide and examined microscopically for the presence of sperm. If present, the percentage of forward (progressive) motility is determined. By definition, this PPM procedure is limited to assessing the presence or absence of sperm and detection of motility. Indications for qualitative semen analysis include initial evaluation of male factor infertility, and post-vasectomy testing. Note that assessment of sperm motility is not an important factor in fertility evaluation unless nearly all sperm are immotile.[16] Routine semen analysis is significantly broader in scope than qualitative semen analysis, and is the test of choice for initial evaluation of male factor infertility.[17]

Clinical Scenario Update

You can perform and interpret the vaginal wet mount procedure yourself if all of the following conditions are met:

- You are a provider (physician, PA, nurse practitioner, nurse midwife, or dentist).
- The clinic laboratory has a valid CLIA certificate for PPM procedures.
- All requirements of PPM procedure testing have been met, including payment of the biannual certificate renewal fee, notification to the state agency within 30 days of any change in laboratory ownership, name, address or director, and allowing on-site inspections by CMS.

As you are a PA and the other conditions have been met, you complete the wet mount, appropriately following all procedures. The results show motile protozoa consistent with trichomonads (Video 1). You diagnose *Trichomonas vaginalis* and decide on a treatment plan with your patient.

SUMMARY

Medial providers practicing in a clinic with the appropriate CLIA certification can perform PPM procedures during clinic visits. Potential benefits include improved quality of care through reduced cost, improved specimen quality, patient convenience, enhanced diagnostic turnaround time, and improved patient satisfaction.

Resources

The author finds the following reference from the Centers for Disease Control and Prevention to be the most comprehensive and practical resource for clinics seeking CLIA PPM procedure certification, providers who perform PPM procedures, and for medical education programs: *Provider-Performed Microscopy Procedures – A Focus on Quality Procedures*.[18] This document includes sections on the background of PPM procedures, relevant regulatory requirements, personnel, safety issues, location for testing, performing PPM procedures, proficiency testing requirements, a quality system description, tips, and resources. The appendices include clear and detailed instructions on the procedure for performing each PPM procedure. The resources section includes CLIA and Health Insurance Portability and Accountability Act links, safety links, and training links, in addition to references.

SUPPLEMENTARY DATA

Supplementary data related to this article can be found online at https://doi.org/10.1016/j.cpha.2019.02.004.

REFERENCES

1. Florkowski C, Don-Wauchope A, Gimenez N, et al. Point-of-care testing (POCT) and evidence-based laboratory medicine (EBLM) - does it leverage any advantage in clinical decision making? Crit Rev Clin Lab Sci 2017;54(7–8):471–94.
2. Asprey D. Clinical skills utilized by physician assistants in rural primary care settings. J Physician Assist Educ 2006;17(2):45–7.
3. Shives T. Testing at a glance: vaginal wet mount. North Carolina State Laboratory of Public Health Technical Bulletin 2016;12(1):104. Available at: https://slph.ncpublichealth.com/doc/TechBulletins/Vol-12-Issue1-wetmount.pdf. Accessed November 2, 2018.
4. Brown GR, Wigdahl JB, Stebens TM. Provider-performed microscopy empowers PAs at the point of care. JAAPA 2018;31(3):19–24.
5. Centers for Medicare and Medicaid Services. Clinical Laboratory Improvements Amendment (CLIA). Available at: https://www.fda.gov/MedicalDevices/DeviceRegulationandGuidance/IVDRegulatoryAssistance/ucm124105.htm. Accessed October 15, 2018.
6. Center for Medicare and Medicaid Services. CLIA categorizations. Available at: https://www.fda.gov/MedicalDevices/DeviceRegulationandGuidance/IVDRegulatoryAssistance/ucm393229.htm. Accessed October 15, 2018.
7. Code of Federal Regulations US Government Publishing Office. Code of Federal Regulations, title 42 – public health, part 493 – laboratory requirements, section 15 laboratories performing waived tests. 2010. Available at: https://www.gpo.gov/fdsys/granule/CFR-2010-title42-vol5/CFR-2010-title42-vol5-sec493-15. Accessed October 15, 2018.
8. US Department of Health & Human Services, US Food & Drug Administration. CLIA—Clinical Laboratory Improvement Amendments—currently waived analytes. Available at: https://www.accessdata.fda.gov/scripts/cdrh/cfdocs/cfClia/analyteswaived.cfm. Accessed November 2, 2018.
9. US Government Printing Office. Code of Federal Regulations, title 42 – public health, part 493 – laboratory requirements, section 19 provider-performed microscopy (PPM) procedures. 2010. Available at: www.gpo.gov/fdsys/granule/CFR-2010-title42-vol5/CFR-2010-title42-vol5-sec493-19. Accessed October 15, 2018.
10. Form CMS-116, Clinical Laboratory Improvement Amendments (CLIA) application for certification. Available at: https://www.cms.gov/Medicare/CMS-Forms/CMS-Forms/downloads/cms116.pdf. Accessed November 2, 2018.
11. Amsel R, Totten PA, Spiegel CA, et al. Nonspecific vaginitis. Diagnostic criteria and microbial and epidemiological associations. Am J Med 1983;74(1):14–22.
12. Stoner KA, Rabe LK, Meyn LA, et al. Survival of Trichomonas vaginalis in wet preparation and on wet mount. Sex Transm Infect 2013;89(6):485–8.
13. Practice Committee of the American Society for Reproductive Medicine. Diagnostic evaluation of the infertile female: a committee opinion. Fertil Steril 2015;103(6):e44.

14. Provider-performed microscopic procedures. Available at: https://www.cms.gov/ Regulations-and-Guidance/Legislation/CLIA/Downloads/ppmplist.pdf. Accessed November 4, 2018.
15. Huicho L, Sanchez D, Contreras M, et al. Occult blood and fecal leukocytes as screening tests in childhood infectious diarrhea: an old problem revisited. Pediatr Infect Dis J 1993;12(6):474.
16. Wang C, Swerdloff RS. Limitations of semen analysis as a test of male fertility and anticipated needs from newer tests. Fertil Steril 2014;102(6):1502.
17. Barratt CLR, Björndahl L, De Jonge CJ, et al. The diagnosis of male infertility: an analysis of the evidence to support the development of global WHO guidance— challenges and future research opportunities. Hum Reprod Update 2017;23(6): 660–80.
18. Provider-performed microscopy procedures—a focus on quality procedures. Available at: https://wwwn.cdc.gov/clia/Resources/PPMP/pdf/15_258020-A_Stang_ PPMP_Booklet_FINAL.pdf. Accessed September 22, 2018.

Immunohematology and Transfusion Medicine

Carey L. Barry, MHS, PA-C, MT(ASCP)

KEYWORDS

- Blood type • ABO blood group • Crossmatch • Type and screen • Blood bank
- Transfusion • Blood products

KEY POINTS

- Blood typing identifies antigens on the membrane of red blood cells to determine the major ABO blood group, Rh type, and other minor blood group antigens.
- Immunohematology remains the foundation of transfusion medicine.
- Although screening and standards improve the safety of blood products, there are inherent risks associated with transfusion.
- Restrictive packed red blood cell transfusion practices are replacing liberal transfusion in most patient populations.

INTRODUCTION

The first successful human blood transfusion was performed by a British obstetrician in 1818; the first description of blood groups was described by Dr Karl Landsteiner in 1900, and crossmatching blood of donor and recipient blood was suggested to improve safety in 1907.[1] Although there have been many improvements and advancements in blood product transfusion, these discoveries remain the foundation of transfusion medicine today. Immunohematology refers to the hematologic antigens found on the membrane of red blood cells (RBCs) and the associated circulating antibodies and is often referred to as blood banking. The antigens of the RBC membranes are composed of carbohydrates and proteins, and the antibodies can be naturally occurring or induced. These antibodies and antigens determine the compatibility of donor blood for transfusion to a recipient.

Disclosure Statement: The author has no disclosures. The author has no relationship with a commercial company that has a direct financial interest in the subject matter or materials discussed in article or with a company making a competing product.
Physician Assistant Program, Bouvé College of Health Sciences, Northeastern University, 202 Robinson Hall, 360 Huntington Avenue, Boston, MA, 02115, USA
E-mail address: c.barry@northeastern.edu

Physician Assist Clin 4 (2019) 591–607
https://doi.org/10.1016/j.cpha.2019.02.009
2405-7991/19/© 2019 Elsevier Inc. All rights reserved.

Blood Type, Antibodies, and Antigens

ABO blood group

The ABO blood group is the most significant in regards to blood and blood product transfusions. There are 4 major blood types: A, B, O, and AB; collectively these are referred to as the ABO blood group. ABO blood group is determined by antigens on the RBC membrane made of carbohydrates. The carbohydrates present on the RBC membrane are created by enzymatic reactions. The foundation or precursor of the ABO group antigens, the H antigen, is present on RBC membranes except for in rare genetic absence.[2] Individuals with type O blood have the H antigen with the absence of A or B antigens. An enzymatic reaction will add the A and B carbohydrate antigens to the H antigen, resulting in type A blood, type B blood, or type AB blood based on which enzymes are present and which antigen or antigens have been added to the H antigen[3] (**Fig. 1**). The enzymes an individual has to form the ABO group are inherited via a Mendelian pattern, whereby the A and B genotypes have a codominance and type O has a recessive pattern[2] (**Fig. 2**).

There are many variations within the ABO blood group. Although the most common variations in the A antigen subtypes are A_1 and A_2, there are many other less common subtypes within the ABO group. For example, the Bombay blood type is a rare genetic variation in which the genotype is hh, and the H antigen is absent on all RBCs.[2] **Fig. 3** includes examples of ABO phenotypes and corresponding genotypes. Type O blood is the most common ABO type in the United States and worldwide with regional and ethnic variation.[2,4] Antibodies of the ABO group are naturally occurring. Individuals with blood type O have naturally occurring anti-A and ant-B antibodies; individuals with blood type A have anti-B antibodies; individuals with blood type B have anti-A antibodies, and individuals with blood type AB have no naturally occurring ABO antibodies[5] (**Fig. 4**, **Table 1**). Individuals with type A_2 can form anti-A_1 antibodies, and individuals with Bombay blood type have anti-H antibodies (see **Table 1**).

Rh blood group

The Rh blood group is determined by antigens made of proteins. The Rh blood system is complex, with 54 possible antigens identified. Although the blood group is named the Rh group, the antigens are not named Rh antigens. The term Rh was initially established after Karl Landsteiner and Alexander Wiener created anti-*rhesus* sera from

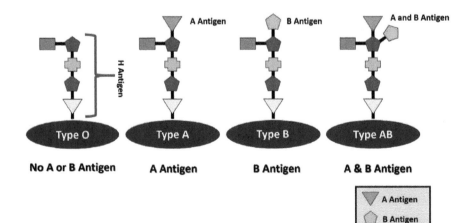

Fig. 1. ABO blood groups with cell membrane antigen types.

Parental Phenotype		B	
	Parental Genotype	B	O
A	A	**AB** *(AB)*	**A** *(AO)*
	O	**B** *(BO)*	**O** *(OO)*

Parental Phenotype	-	Parental Genotype	-	Offspring **Phenotype** *(Genotype)*

Fig. 2. ABO blood groups inheritance pattern.

rabbit serum after injecting the rabbits with rhesus monkey RBCs and discovering that the anti-rhesus sera caused agglutination with human blood cells.[6,7] It was later discovered that the antigen was not the same in humans as in animals; the animal antigen was named LW after Landsteiner and Wiener,[2] and the human Rh antigen was named D antigen. The D antigen was the first Rh antigen discovered, is the most immunogenic, and has the greatest clinical significance.[2,5] Although less significant Rh antigens are known (for example, C, c, E, and e),[2] the Rh designation refers only to the presence or absence of the D antigen. Importantly, unlike ABO antibodies, anti-D antibodies are not naturally occurring, but can be induced because of D antigen exposure.

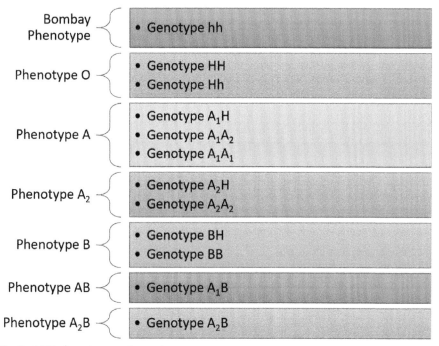

Bombay Phenotype
- Genotype hh

Phenotype O
- Genotype HH
- Genotype Hh

Phenotype A
- Genotype A_1H
- Genotype A_1A_2
- Genotype A_1A_1

Phenotype A_2
- Genotype A_2H
- Genotype A_2A_2

Phenotype B
- Genotype BH
- Genotype BB

Phenotype AB
- Genotype A_1B

Phenotype A_2B
- Genotype A_2B

Fig. 3. ABO phenotype and genotype.

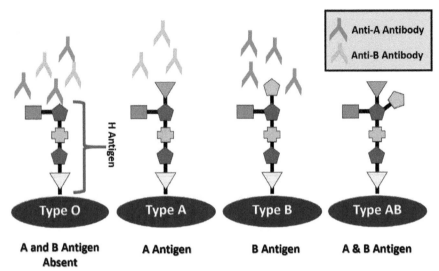

Fig. 4. ABO blood groups antigens with naturally occurring ABO antibodies.

Other blood groups

There are many other minor surface antigens on RBCs (**Box 1**).[2,5,3] Antibodies to these other antigens are not naturally occurring and require exposure to foreign RBC antigens to form the antibodies. Antigens of the other minor types can be problematic if an individual who is negative for an antigen is exposed via blood transfusion and forms antibodies to that antigen. Once antibodies are formed, subsequent transfusions will need to have special donor unit screening for the offending antigen type.

Initially, names for blood groups were labeled alphabetically or according to the individual who was first discovered to have produced the antibodies. The International Society of Blood Transfusion has developed a system that labels each blood group with a 3-digit number in order of discovery and each subgroup within the system is labeled with a 3-digit number after the decimal point of the system number. An example is type B blood, which is 001.002; the first 3 digits (001) refer to the ABO group and the second 3 digits (002) refer to the blood type B. Although this terminology is not commonly used to describe the ABO blood group, it is helpful in the description of the many other RBC membrane antigens that have been identified.

Laboratory Testing

Although serologic immunohematologic testing is sufficient to determine blood type in most cases, molecular testing can be performed to identify blood type if serologic

Table 1			
ABO blood groups, antigens, and antibodies			
ABO Blood Type (Phenotype)	ABO Blood Type (Genotype)	ABO Antigens	ABO Antibodies (Naturally Occurring)
O	OO (HH or Hh)	H	Anti-A and anti-B
A	AO or AA	A	Anti-B
B	BO or BB	B	Anti-A
AB	AB	A and B	None
Bombay	hh	No ABO antigens	Anti-H, anti-A, and anti-B

| Box 1 |
| Blood systems |
| This is a list of a few of the identified blood group systems. Each system has several subtypes. These blood types are relevant but less important than ABO and Rh groups for blood transfusion. |
| Lewis |
| Duffy |
| Diego |
| MNS |
| Lutheran |
| Kidd |
| Kell |
| PIPK |
| Scianna |
| Dombrock |
| Colton |
| Landsteiner-Wiener |
| Chido/Rodgers |

testing is inconclusive, that is, results in a weak hemagglutination reaction. The tube testing method is a reliable and commonly used method of testing for blood type.[8] The sample to be tested is collected and labeled: *patient samples* are collected and labeled with a unique blood bank number that is on the sample and the patient's blood bank or identification band, and as per institution protocol, *donor samples* are labeled in accordance with federal regulations.[9] RBCs from the patient sample are then separated and used to create a sample red cell suspension, and patient serum or plasma is separated for testing (**Fig. 5**). The sample RBCs and serum are then tested with a panel of reagents with known antisera (forward typing), and the sample serum or plasma is tested with a panel of reagent RBCs with known antigens (reverse typing) (**Fig. 6**). After the sample and each reagent are mixed in individually labeled test tubes, the tubes are centrifuged to form a button of red cells at the bottom of the tube. The tubes are then gently agitated to remove the button of red cells at the bottom of the tube, and the degree of clumping is graded (**Fig. 7**). The degree of clumping is graded from 0 to 4: 0 is negative with no clumping and 4 is a solid button of clumping. Some of the more common studies in immunohematologic testing are included in **Table 2** with the common order and what is typically included.

ABO and Rh blood type

ABO blood group is determined via forward typing (sample RBCs) and reverse typing (sample serum or plasma). Rh type is determined with forward typing using the anti-D reagent. In forward typing, the sample RBC suspension is tested with anti-A, anti-B, and anti-D reagent. Reverse typing is performed by adding sample serum or plasma to known A_1 blood cell reagent and B blood cell reagent. The pattern of agglutination in blood typing will indicate the blood type (**Table 3**). If there are weak reactions or a discrepancy with determining the blood type, subtypes must be considered, and further testing must be considered. If further serologic investigation is not able to

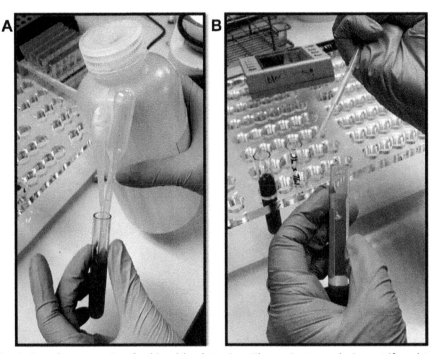

Fig. 5. Sample preparation for blood bank testing: The patient sample is centrifuged to separate the RBCs and the serum or plasma component of the sample. (*A*) Patient RBCs are mixed with normal saline to create an RBC suspension. (*B*) Patient plasma is separated.

identify the blood type, molecular testing could be considered. Type-compatible blood must be used for transfusions of human blood products (**Table 4**).

Antibody screen
The antibody screen is performed by mixing patient serum or plasma with reagent RBCs that have a known panel of antigens comprising many of the non-ABO and non-Rh blood types. This antibody screen will test to see if the patient has formed antibodies to these RBC antigens. If the antibody screen is positive, the antibody will need to be identified with an antibody identification panel. In addition, any blood to be transfused will need to be tested for the antigen or blood type for which the patient has the antibodies, and if present, this blood sample should not be transfused. For example, if a patient tests positive for an anti-Kell antibody, any units with a Kell antigen cannot be transfused. Finding compatible blood when a patient has a positive antibody screen could be more time consuming and more difficult.

Crossmatch
Crossmatching is accomplished by mixing patient's serum with donor RBCs to observe for incompatibility (**Fig. 8**). If there is agglutination when this is performed, it indicates that the recipient may have circulating antibodies to an antigen on the donor RBCs. It will not identify antibodies or antigens present, but serve as an overall screen for compatibility.

Coombs test
Sensitized RBCs are cells that are coated with antibodies (**Fig. 9**). A direct Coombs test or direct antiglobulin test, commonly called Coombs test, is performed to

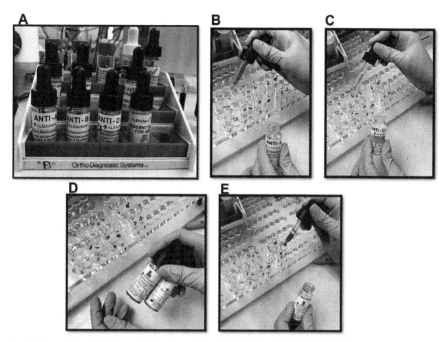

Fig. 6. Blood type testing. (*A*) To determine blood type, patient samples are tested with a panel of reagents that contain antibodies to specific antigens and RBCs that have known antigens for hemagglutination. Patient RBCs are mixed with normal saline to create an RBC suspension, and serum or plasma is separated. (*B, C*) Forward typing is when patient RBC suspension is mixed with reagents with known antibodies and (*D, E*) reverse typing is when patient plasma is tested against a panel of RBCs with known antigens.

determine if the patient's RBCs are sensitized and can be useful to identify antibody-related transfusion reactions. The red cells can be tested for both antibodies and complement coating the cells. Identifying if RBCs are coated with antibodies, compliment, or both antibodies and compliment can be useful to help diagnose a transfusion reaction or other hemolytic processes.

Donor Blood Products and Transfusion

Individuals can donate whole blood, platelets, RBCs, and granulocytes for allogenic transfusion. Whole blood contains all the elements of circulating blood, including erythrocytes, leukocytes, thrombocytes, and plasma. Blood products can be collected as whole blood that is separated into components (RBCs, plasma, and platelets) or via apheresis. Apheresis donation is accomplished by removing blood from the donor and passing the whole blood through an apparatus with a centrifuge or filter to separate out the specific component to be collected, and the remainder of the blood is returned to the donor's circulation. Platelets, plasma, and RBCs can be collected via apheresis. Whole blood can be donated once every 56 days, and platelets can be donated every 7 days up to 24 times a year.

Whole blood

Although whole blood is the most commonly donated blood product, it is rarely transfused as whole blood, and there are no current guidelines or clinical data to support whole blood transfusion.[10] Approximately 450 to 500 mL of whole blood is collected

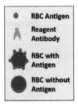

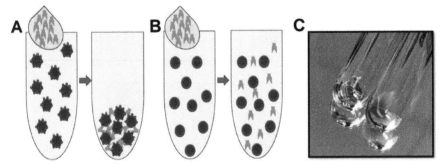

Fig. 7. Hemagglutination testing: Patient RBCs are suspended in normal saline (RBC suspension); then a reagent with antibodies against the antigen being tested (reagent) is added to the RBC suspension. If the antigen is present, the RBCs in the suspension agglutinate. (*A*) RBCs with antigen: Reagent plus RBC suspension results in hemagglutination, (*B*) RBCs without antigen: Reagent plus RBC suspension does not result in hemagglutination, (*C*) image of test tubes with hemagglutination and without hemagglutination. The test tube to the left reflects RBCs with antigen (**Fig. 7**A), and the test tube to the right reflects RBCs without antigen (**Fig.7**B). The reaction strength can be graded.

from the donor and separated into components for transfusion. One unit of whole blood can be separated into packed red blood cells (PRBC), plasma, and platelets. The unit of whole blood is centrifuged with a soft spin and separated into PRBCs and platelet-rich plasma (PRP); then, the PRP is centrifuged with a hard spin separating into a platelet concentrate and fresh plasma that is frozen to create fresh frozen plasma (FFP) (**Fig. 10**).[5]

Packed red blood cells
PRBC are one of the most used blood products. Each unit contains approximately 300 to 400 mL total volume with an estimated hematocrit (Hct) of 55% to 65% in

Table 2
Immunohematology laboratory studies

Laboratory Order	Testing Included
ABO blood type	ABO type
Rh blood type	Rh type
Blood type	ABO type, Rh type
Antibody screen	Antibody screen
Type and screen	ABO type, Rh type, antibody screen
Crossmatch (number of units)	Crossmatch
Type and cross (number of units)	ABO, Rh, antibody screen, crossmatch
Transfuse (product & units)	Transfusion of type and crossed units
Coombs test (direct or indirect)	Coombs test

Table 3
Blood type testing: hemagglutination testing for blood type

Reagent Blood Type	Anti-A	Anti-B	Anti-D	A_1 Cell Suspension	B Cell Suspension
A positive	+	−	+	−	+
A negative	+	−	−	−	+
B positive	−	+	+	+	−
B negative	−	+	−	+	−
AB positive	+	+	+	−	−
AB negative	+	+	−	−	−
O positive	−	−	+	+	+
O negative	−	−	−	+	+

Abbreviations: +, agglutination; −, no agglutination.

Table 4
Blood product compatibility

Recipient Blood Type	Antigens	Antibodies	Compatible PRBCs	Compatible FFP	Compatible Platelets
O+	H	Anti-A Anti-B	O+ O−	O A B AB	O+ preferred O− A+ A− B+ B− AB+ AB−
O−	H	Anti-A Anti-B	O−	O A B AB	O− preferred A− B− AB−
A+	A	Anti-B	O+ O− A+ A−	A AB	A+ preferred A− AB+ AB−
A−	A	Anti-B	O− A−	A AB	A− preferred AB−
B+	B	Anti-A	O+ O− B+ B−	B AB	B+ preferred B− AB+ AB−
B−	B	Anti-A	O− B−	B AB	B− preferred AB−
AB+	A & B	None	O+ O− A+ A− B+ B− AB+ AB−	AB	AB+ preferred AB−
AB−	A & B	None	O− A− B− AB−	AB	AB− preferred

Type O− is the universal PRBC donor; type AB is the universal FFP donor; type AB+ is the universal PRBC recipient; and type O is the universal FFP recipient.

A

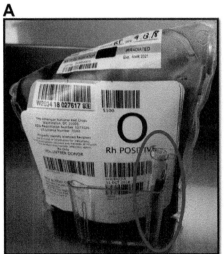

B

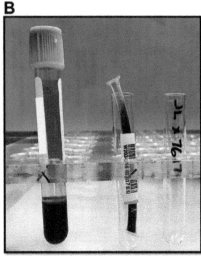

Fig. 8. Crossmatch: Donor units are prepared with tubing that contains donor blood and has been crimped in multiple small segments to be used for testing. (*A*) Donor unit with tubing to be used for testing (circled in red). (*B*) A crossmatch will be performed by mixing recipient serum with donor RBCs. If there is no clumping, the unit is considered compatible; any clumping would indicate the unit is not compatible and should not be transfused to the patient.

preservative solution, anticoagulant, and 20 to 100 mL of donor plasma.[3,10–12] The shelf life of PRBCs is 42 days when refrigerated and up to 10 years if frozen within 6 days of collection. Cryoprotective agents must be removed from frozen PRBC units before transfusion.[12] One unit of PRBC is expected to increase the hemoglobin (Hgb) concentration by 1 g/dL and the Hct by 3% (**Table 5**), and the Hgb and Hct typically equilibrate about 15 minutes after receiving the transfusion.[11,13]

RBCs can be treated in several different ways: washed, leukoreduced, and irradiated. *Washed RBCs* are washed with a solution that will remove almost all of the plasma and decrease the number of platelets and leukocytes; however, there is some associated RBC loss with washing. After washing, the PRBC unit has a shelf life of 24 hours because of the need to enter the sealed unit container.[11] Leukocytes contained in PRBC and platelet units for transfusion are associated with adverse effects, including febrile nonhemolytic reaction, bacterial infections, cytomegalovirus infection, and graft-versus-host disease.[3,11] Leukoreduction of RBCs can improve the risk of some these effects. Currently, leukoreduction filters are used and are effective. *Irradiated PRBC* are treated with a dose of radiation to kill all the leukocytes and are the most effective way to eliminate the risk of graft-versus-host disease in severely immunocompromised patients or patients undergoing chemotherapy. *Indications for PRBC transfusion* have had some recent changes. Literature supports a restrictive approach to transfusion using a threshold Hgb of between 7 g/dL and 8 g/dL, and studies have shown equivalent outcomes with decreased blood product utilization.[14–19] The restrictive approach in patients with known coronary artery disease and acute coronary syndrome is not clear with some conflicting data and a lack of a multicenter randomized control trial.[18,20–23] The most recent American Association of Blood Banks (AABB) guidelines recommend a threshold of 7 g/dL for hemodynamically stable hospitalized adults, including critically ill, and a restrictive threshold of 8 g/

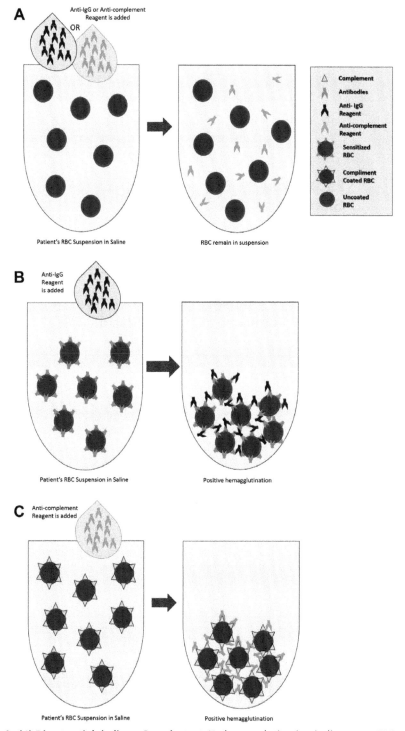

Fig. 9. (*A*) **Direct antiglobulin or Coombs test**: No hemagglutination indicates no RBC sensitization; Coombs test is negative. (*B*) **Direct antiglobulin or Coombs test**: Hemagglutination indicates the patient's RBCs are sensitized; Coombs test is positive. (*C*) **Positive Coombs test for complement**: Hemagglutination indicates the patients RBCs are coated with complement; Coombs test is positive for complement. IgG, immunoglobulin G.

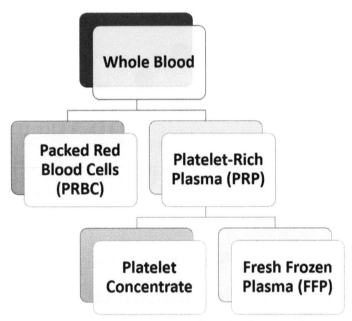

Fig. 10. Component separation: Whole blood is collected and separated into 3 components: PRBC, platelet concentrate, and FFP.

dL is recommended for patients undergoing orthopedic surgery, patients undergoing cardiac surgery, and patients with preexisting cardiac disease.[24,25] Transfusion of PRBC must be with compatible blood types (see **Table 4**).

Platelets

Platelets can be concentrated from whole blood or collected via apheresis. Platelet concentrates from whole blood can be pooled to increase the number of platelets for transfusion. The disadvantage is the increase of donor exposure to about 5 to 10 pooled platelet concentrates compared with single donor exposure with an apheresis pack. Indications for platelet transfusion include a threshold platelet count less than 10,000/μL or less than 5000/μL if the patient has no fevers or infections. The target platelet count for small procedures (central venous catheter, lumbar puncture,

Table 5
Blood products: volume and expected outcome from transfusion of 1 unit

Blood Product Component	Volume, mL	Expected Outcome
PRBC	~300	↑ Hgb 1 g/dL or ↑ Hct 3% per unit
FFP	~200	↓ PT/INR, PTT
Platelet pheresis pack	~250	↑ 10,0000–60,000/μL
Platelet concentrate	~50	↑ 5000–10,000/μL

Abbreviations: Hgb, hemoglobin; Hct, hematocrit; INR, international normalized ratio; PT, prothrombin time; PTT, partial thromboplastin time.

or bone marrow biopsy) is 20,000/μL. The target level in preparing for surgery or invasive procedures is 50,000/μL.[10,12] Platelet transfusion is always considered with active hemorrhage (**Box 2**). Platelet transfusion has also been shown to decrease need for PRBC with massive transfusions in trauma patients.[26]

Fresh frozen plasma
Plasma can be concentrated from whole blood or collected via apheresis (plasmapheresis). A concentrate from whole blood will contain a volume of about 200 to 250 mL, whereas plasmapheresis typically contains a volume of 400 to 600 mL.[3,10] Fresh plasma must be frozen within 6 hours of collection, and once thawed, can be stored for 5 days when refrigerated or 8 hours at room temperature. FFP contains coagulation factors, and the half-life of the factors should be considered when determining timing of transfusion. For example, when transfusing to correct coagulopathy before surgery, the FFP should be administered within a few hours of surgery as opposed to the day before. Indications for transfusion are correction of coagulopathy or active bleeding. Coagulation studies can be used to monitor correction of coagulopathy.

Transfusion Safety and Risks

Donor blood testing and safety
The safety, collection, processing, and administration of human blood and blood products are regulated by the US Food and Drug Administration (FDA) and guidelines set forth by the Centers for Disease Control and Prevention (CDC).[9,12,27] Ensuring safety in transfusion of human products begins with donor screening and donor unit testing. Donors are screened for general health, medical conditions, sexually transmitted disease, medical treatments, medications, vaccinations, travel, and lifestyle and life events. In addition, donated blood undergoes testing for blood type and antibodies as well as infectious disease testing.[10,12] The World Health Organization

---

Box 2
Indication for blood product transfusion

Packed Red Blood Cells

- Threshold of Hgb less than 7 g/dL hemodynamically stable hospitalized adults
- Threshold of less than 8 g/dL in patients undergoing orthopedic surgery, cardiac surgery, and patients with preexisting cardiac disease
- Severe symptoms of anemia
- Active hemorrhage

Platelets

- Threshold platelet count less than 10,000/μL
- Threshold of less than 5000/μL may be sufficient without fever or infections
- 20,000/μL target level for central venous catheter
- 50,000/μL target level for invasive procedures
- Active hemorrhage

Fresh Frozen Plasma

- Correction of coagulopathy
- Rapid correction of warfarin
- Active hemorrhage

recommends blood grouping and compatibility testing as well as infectious testing for human immunodeficiency virus (HIV), hepatitis B, hepatitis C, and syphilis.[28] In addition to blood type, infectious testing for the following is required by the CDC: bacterial contamination, hepatitis B virus, hepatitis C virus, HIV types 1 and 2, human T-lymphotropic virus, syphilis, and West Nile virus.[27] The American Red Cross provides much of the blood product supply in the United States.[29] In addition to the required testing as indicated by the CDC, the American Red Cross currently screens for Chagas disease, Zika virus, select regional screening for babesiosis, and select cytomegalovirus screening.[30]

Despite screening and testing processes, there are still risks associated with human blood product transfusion. Specific measures are required to help minimize risk of adverse reactions (**Box 3**).

Adverse reactions to blood transfusion can be divided into 4 major categories: acute immunologic reactions, delayed immunologic reactions, acute nonimmunologic reactions, and delayed nonimmunologic reactions[3,10] (**Box 4**). Before receiving a transfusion, patients need to be informed of the risks associated with receiving transfusion as well as the alternatives to blood product transfusion (**Box 4**). In addition, patients must be monitored closely for adverse reactions and promptly treated for complications that arise.

Autologous and Directed Blood Products

Autologous donation is when a patient donates blood for him- or herself, and directed donation is when an individual donates blood for a specific patient with a compatible blood type. Both autologous and directed units of blood and blood products will be

---

Box 3
Specific measures that need to be taken to improve safety of blood transfusions

- Mix units thoroughly and visually inspect for abnormalities
- Follow institution protocol to identify recipient and confirm intended unit
- Use aseptic techniques for transfusion
- Transfuse through 150- to 260-μn filter to remove clots and aggregates
- Warm units with FDA-approved warming device if clinically indicated (ie, massive transfusion or cold-reactive antibodies)
- Complete transfusion within 4 hours if the unit is kept at room temperature (24 hours if refrigerated)
- Do not infuse medications or lactated Ringer or calcium containing solution in the same tubing
- Slow infusion to monitor for reactions unless rapid infusion is clinically indicated
- Monitoring and recording vital signs before, during, and after transfusion
- Discontinue transfusion immediately if transfusion reaction suspected
- Report all suspected bacterial contamination and transfusion-related infectious disease transmission
- Consider voluntary reporting of transfusion-related adverse events to National Healthcare Safety Network at https://www.cdc.gov/nhsn/acute-care-hospital/bio-hemo/

Data from Bachowski G, Borge D, Brunker P, et al. A compendium of transfusion practice guidelines. 3rd edition. Washington, DC: American Red Cross. 2017. Available at: https://www.redcrossblood.org/content/dam/redcrossblood/documents/transfusionpractices-compendium_3rdedition.pdf. Accessed November 10, 2018.

Box 4
Adverse transfusion reactions: 4 categories of transfusion reactions include acute immunologic reactions, delayed immunologic reactions, acute nonimmunologic reactions, and delayed nonimmunologic reactions

Acute Immunologic Reactions

- Febrile transfusion reaction
- Transfusion-related acute lung injury
- Allergic
- Acute hemolytic transfusion reaction

Delayed Immunologic Reactions

- Delayed hemolytic transfusion reaction
- Posttransfusion purpura

Acute Nonimmunologic Reactions

- Transfusion associated circulatory overload
- Citrate toxicity
- Hypothermia
- Bacterial contamination

Delayed nonimmunologic reactions

- Infectious disease

---

donated and processed in the same manner as all other donated blood products, including blood typing, antibody screening, and infectious disease testing. After screening and processing, the blood products will be transferred to the local blood bank where the patient will receive care. Patients receiving autologous and directed donation transfusions undergo the same testing and processing as they would to receive any blood product transfusion. Testing and processing includes blood typing, antibody screening, crossmatch, and the patient identification processes specific to transfusion. An example of potential use of autologous donation is in preparation for surgery. A patient will typically donate blood about a month before surgery to allow the blood time to be processed, to allow the blood product to be viable for transfusion, and for the patient to have time to regenerate circulating volume of blood. Autologous and directed donation can be useful for individuals with a rare blood type or with antibodies.

SUMMARY

The understanding of immunohematology had drastically improved over the last century, but the fundamental principles have remained the same. Although transfusion medicine has lifesaving potential, as with many aspects of medicine, it remains a balance of risk versus benefit. With the recent changes to a more restrictive PRBC transfusion practice, patient benefit has remained steady and need for transfusion has decreased. Still, further studies are needed in the areas of restrictive and liberal transfusion practices in the patient population with acute coronary syndrome and traumatic brain injury.

REFERENCES

1. AABB. Highlights of transfusion medicine history. Available at: http://www.aabb.org/tm/Pages/highlights.aspx. Accessed November 4, 2018.

2. Daniels G. Human blood groups. In: ProQuest, editor. 3rd edition. Chichester (West Sussex): John Wiley & Sons; 2013.

3. Dzieczkowski JS, Tiberghien P, Anderson KC. Transfusion Biology and Therapy. In: Jameson J, Fauci AS, Kasper DL, Hauser SL, Longo DL, Loscalzo J. eds. Harrison's Principles of Internal Medicine, 20e. New York, NY: McGraw-Hill; http://accessmedicine.mhmedical.com/content.aspx?bookid=2129&sectionid=192280 223. Accessed April 01, 2019.

4. Garratty G, Glynn SA, McEntire R. ABO and Rh(D) phenotype frequencies of different racial/ ethnic groups in the United States. Transfusion 2004;44(5):703–6.

5. Franklin Bunn H. Pathophysiology of blood disorders 2nd edition. In: Pathophysiology of blood disorders, 2e. 2nd edition. Mcgraw-Hill Education; 2017.

6. Landsteiner K, Wiener AS. An agglutinable factor in human blood recognized by immune sera for rhesus blood. Proc Soc Exp Biol Med 1940;43(1):223.

7. Landsteiner K, Wiener AS. Studies on an agglutinogen (Rh) in human blood reacting with anti-rhesus sera and with human isoantibodies. J Exp Med 1941; 74(4):309.

8. Mujahid A, Dickert FL. Blood group typing: from classical strategies to the application of synthetic antibodies generated by molecular imprinting. Sensors (Basel, Switzerland) 2015;16(1):51.

9. Title 21, US Code of Federal Regulations, Section 606. 1(f): Current Good Manufacturing Practice for Blood and Blood Components. In: Administration USFD, ed. p. 21.

10. Bachowski G, Borge D, Brunker P, et al. A compendium of transfusion practice guidelines. 3rd edition. Washington, DC: American Red Cross; 2017. Available at: https://www.redcrossblood.org/content/dam/redcrossblood/documents/transfusionpractices-compendium_3rdedition.pdf. Accessed November 10, 2018.

11. McCullough J. Transfusion medicine. Chicester (United Kingdom): John Wiley & Sons, Incorporated; 2011.

12. Center for Biologics, Evaluation Research. AABB, American Red Cross, America's Blood Centers, Armed Services Blood Program. Guidance for industry an acceptable circular of information for the use of human blood and blood components. Acceptable circular of information for the use of human blood and blood components 2003. Available at: http://www.aabb.org/tm/coi/Pages/default.aspx. Accessed November 12, 2018.

13. Wiesen AR, Hospenthal DR, Byrd JC, et al. Equilibration of hemoglobin concentration after transfusion in medical inpatients not actively bleeding. Ann Intern Med 1994;121(4):278.

14. Holst LB, Petersen MW, Haase N, et al. Restrictive versus liberal transfusion strategy for red blood cell transfusion: systematic review of randomised trials with meta-analysis and trial sequential analysis. BMJ 2015;350:h1354.

15. Parker MJ. Randomised trial of blood transfusion versus a restrictive transfusion policy after hip fracture surgery. Injury 2013;44(12):1916–8.

16. Roubinian N, Carson JL. Red blood cell transfusion strategies in adult and pediatric patients with malignancy. Hematol Oncol Clin North Am 2016;30(3):529–40.

17. Hayes M, Uhl L. To transfuse or not transfuse: an intensive appraisal of red blood cell transfusions in the ICU. Curr Opin Hematol 2018;25(6):468–72.

18. Mazer CD, Whitlock RP, Fergusson DA, et al. Restrictive or liberal red-cell transfusion for cardiac surgery. N Engl J Med 2017;377(22):2133–44.

19. Hebert PC, Wells G, Blajchman MA, et al. A multicenter, randomized, controlled clinical trial of transfusion requirements in critical care. N Engl J Med 1999;340(6):409–17.

20. Koch CG, Li L, Sessler DI, et al. Duration of red-cell storage and complications after cardiac surgery. N Engl J Med 2008;358(12):1229–39.

21. Carson JL, Brooks MM, Abbott JD, et al. Liberal versus restrictive transfusion thresholds for patients with symptomatic coronary artery disease. Am Heart J 2013;165(6):964–71.e1.

22. Garfinkle M, Lawler PR, Filion KB, et al. Red blood cell transfusion and mortality among patients hospitalized for acute coronary syndromes: a systematic review. Int J Cardiol 2013;164(2):151–7.

23. Cortes-Puch I, Wiley B, Sun J, et al. Risks of restrictive red blood cell transfusion strategies in patients with cardiovascular disease (CVD): a meta-analysis. Transfus Med 2018;28(5):335–45.

24. Carson JL, Guyatt G, Heddle NM, et al. Clinical practice guidelines from the AABB: red blood cell transfusion thresholds and storage. JAMA 2016;316(19):2025–35.

25. Yazer MH, Triulzi DJ. AABB red blood cell transfusion guidelines: something for almost everyone. JAMA 2016;316(19):1984.

26. Hallet J, Lauzier F, Mailloux O, et al. The use of higher platelet:RBC transfusion ratio in the acute phase of trauma resuscitation: a systematic review. Crit Care Med 2013;41(12):2800–11.

27. Centers for Disease Control and Prevention (CDC). Blood safety basics. Available at: https://www.cdc.gov/bloodsafety/basics.html. Accessed November 07, 2018.

28. The World Health Organization. Blood safety and avalability fact sheet. Available at: http://www.who.int/en/news-room/fact-sheets/detail/blood-safety-and-availability. Accessed November 4, 2018.

29. Institute of Medicine (US) Committee to Study HIV Transmission Through Blood and Blood Products. HIV and the blood supply: an analysis of crisis decisionmaking. In: Leveton LB, SHJ, Stoto MA, editors. HIV and the blood supply: an analysis of crisis decisionmaking. National Academies Press (US); 1995.

30. The American Red Cross. Infectious disease testing. 2018. Available at: https://www.redcrossblood.org/biomedical-services/blood-diagnostic-testing/blood-testing.html. Accessed November 11, 2018.

Laboratory Evaluation of Hemostasis Disorders

Mary Jean Leonardi, MAT, MMS, PA-C

KEYWORDS

- Hemostasis • Coagulation cascade • Bleeding disorder • Thrombophilia
- Anticoagulation monitoring

KEY POINTS

- Disruptions in the normal process of hemostasis can give rise to either disorders of bleeding or disorders of clotting.
- Evaluation of a patient with a complaint of excessive bleeding begins with a detailed and focused history and physical examination.
- Laboratory evaluation of a patient with excessive bleeding begins with basic laboratory studies, including a complete blood count (CBC), peripheral blood smear, complete metabolic panel (CMP), and coagulation laboratory studies including prothrombin time (PT), activated partial thromboplastin time (aPTT), and/or thrombin time (TT).
- Extensive laboratory testing is available to assess causes of genetic or acquired thrombophilia, but is only indicated in specific circumstances.
- Laboratory tests that help identify underlying disorders can also be used to monitor the level of anticoagulation medications.

INTRODUCTION

Hemostasis is the process by which bleeding from a blood vessel is stopped. It involves a complex system of positive and negative feedback processes to promote rapid clot formation in areas where the integrity of a blood vessel is compromised while limiting the size of the clot and allowing for dissolution of the clot as the vessel wall is repaired. Disruptions to this system can cause either excessive bleeding (hemophilia) or excessive/inappropriate clot formation (thrombophilia). This article examines the normal physiologic process and where disruptions can occur, and describes the laboratory diagnostics available to evaluate the underlying causes in a patient with either hemophilia or thrombophilia.

Disclosure Statement: Nothing to disclose.
Physician Assistant Program, Department of PA Studies, Wake Forest School of Medicine, Medical Center Boulevard, Winston-Salem, NC 27157-1006, USA
E-mail address: maleonar@wakehealth.edu

Physician Assist Clin 4 (2019) 609–623
https://doi.org/10.1016/j.cpha.2019.02.014
2405-7991/19/© 2019 Elsevier Inc. All rights reserved.

HEMOSTASIS

The process of hemostasis involves several steps (**Fig. 1**). First, damage to the endo-thelial wall of a blood vessel exposes cell membranes and their surface proteins, including collagen and tissue factor (TF). The damage to the vessel wall induces vaso-constriction to help limit the loss of blood from the vessel. Next, nearby platelets become activated and aggregate at the site of damage. Simultaneously, proteins (coagulation factors) found in the blood are activated to promote the production of fibrin, a "sticky" protein that helps bind aggregated platelets to each other and the blood vessel wall, forming a clot. Finally, other proteins are activated simultaneously that inhibit clot formation to prevent the clot from growing too large. The process of fibri-nolysis is also initiated to promote dissolution of the clot as the vessel wall is repaired.[1,2]

PLATELET ACTIVATION/AGGREGATION

Platelets are small, nonnucleated cells formed in the bone marrow from large progen-itor cells called megakaryocytes. They are released into the peripheral blood and circulate approximately 10 days.[3] When the endothelium of a blood vessel is damaged, collagen molecules in the underlying connective tissue layers are exposed. Platelet receptors can bind directly to collagen, but binding is enhanced via an inter-mediary molecule named von Willebrand factor (vWF).[2,4] Binding triggers a complex series of changes inside the platelet. Ultimately, the changes alter the intracellular matrix, inducing a shape change from more rounded to flattened with multiple pseu-dopods. Additionally, binding of platelets to collagen promotes extracellular release of molecules from several different types of granules, including dense granules and α granules.[4] Some of the molecules, including serotonin and ADP, help to promote acti-vation of nearby platelets. Other molecules, such as vWF and fibrinogen, help to pro-mote aggregation and binding of platelets to each other at the site of damage.[4] Additionally, activated platelets upregulate molecules on their cell membranes that promote activation of the coagulation cascade.[2,4]

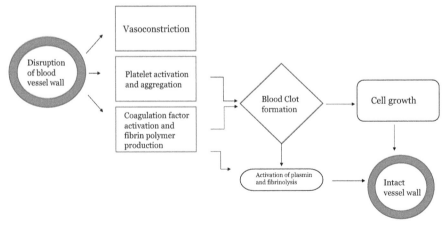

Fig. 1. Mechanisms of hemostasis. Hemostasis mechanisms include vasoconstriction to reduce blood loss, platelet activation and aggregation to form a platelet plug at the area of damage, and activation of the coagulation cascade to form fibrin polymers that are cross-linked to form a stable clot. Activation of the coagulation cascade also activates the process of fibrinolysis that slowly dissolves the clot as cell growth is stimulated under it, leading to an intact blood vessel wall.

COAGULATION CASCADE

Ultimately, the coagulation cascade produces cross-linked fibrin proteins that form a meshwork to bind platelet aggregates into a cohesive unit. As the process of coagulation was being unraveled, the various molecules were called "factors" and were often named after the patient in which a deficiency was recognized (eg, Christmas factor, Stuart-Prower factor).[5] The nomenclature for coagulation molecules was standardized in the 1960s. Molecules were still called "factors" but were given Roman numeral designations (eg, factor I, factor II).[5] These factors were found to be held in inactive forms in the blood, and would be modified into active forms. The active forms were therefore designated with an "a" after the Roman numeral (eg, II vs IIa, X vs Xa).[6]

In vitro analysis of the coagulation cascade led to the view of two separately activated pathways (intrinsic and extrinsic) that converge in a common pathway that yields the production of fibrin (**Fig. 2**).[2] In vivo analysis, however, has given rise to an integrated model where the factors associated with the extrinsic pathway initiate the formation of thrombin, whereas the factors associated with the intrinsic pathway and activated platelets help to propagate and amplify the process.[6–9] In laboratory testing, it is still useful to look at the historical, in vitro model to help evaluate results. Therefore, this article looks in more detail at the in vitro model.[2,10,11]

Extrinsic Pathway

The extrinsic pathway involves activation of factor X via Tissue Factor (TF) and factor VII. TF is found on cell membranes of cells not normally exposed to blood, such as smooth muscle cells. When there is endothelial damage, TF is exposed. TF binds to factor VII and forms factor VIIa. The TF/VIIa complex then activates factor X, which is the beginning of the common pathway (see **Fig. 2A**).

Intrinsic Pathway

The intrinsic pathway involves factors VIII, IX, XI, and XII. In vitro, it is initiated when factor XII contacts negatively charged molecules that causes the formation of factor

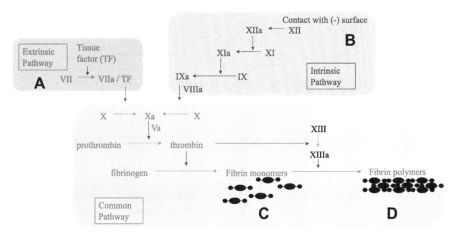

Fig. 2. Coagulation cascade. The coagulation cascade in vitro includes the extrinsic (A) and intrinsic (B) pathways that converge in the formation of factor Xa. In the common pathway, thrombin cleaves fibrinogen to form fibrin monomers (C). The monomers are cross-linked into polymers by factor XIIIa. The polymers help stabilize the platelet aggregate, forming a clot (D).

XIIa. Factor XIIa then activates factor XI, forming factor XIa. Factor XIa then activates factor IX, forming factor IXa. Factor IXa forms a complex with factor VIIIa that activates factor X (see **Fig. 2**B).

Common Pathway

The difference between the intrinsic and extrinsic pathways is how factor Xa is produced. Once produced, factor Xa combines with factor Va to form prothrombinase. This complex acts on prothrombin (factor II) to form thrombin. Thrombin (factor IIa) then modifies fibrinogen (factor I) into fibrin monomers (see **Fig. 2**C). Activated factor XIII (XIIIa) then cross-links monomers to form fibrin polymers (see **Fig. 2**D).

INHIBITORY MOLECULES AND FIBRINOLYSIS

Multiple processes are used to limit clot formation. This helps prevent inappropriate clot formation in areas without damage, and limits the size of clots to prevent stenosis of the blood vessel. Some of these molecules, such as protein C and antithrombin, work to convert activated factors into inactive molecules. Other molecules, such as plasmin, directly cleave fibrin polymers (**Fig. 3**).

Inhibitory Molecules

Protein C is an inhibitory molecule found in the blood. It is converted to an active form by a thrombin-thrombomodulin complex. Activated protein C binds with its cofactor, protein S, to form a complex that converts factor XIIIa and factor Va into inactive forms, thus blunting clot formation (see **Fig. 3**A).[12,13] Additionally, activated protein C seems to help modulate inflammation and maintain the integrity of the endothelial barrier.[14]

Antithrombin is another inhibitory molecule found in the blood. It binds to multiple activated factors, but primarily forms an irreversible bond with thrombin (factor IIa) and with factor Xa that inactivates those factors (see **Fig. 3**B).[12]

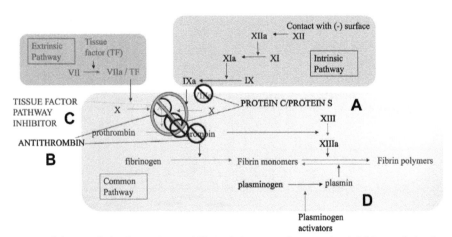

Fig. 3. Inhibitors of clot formation and fibrinolysis. Naturally occurring inhibitors of clot formation help limit the size of clots. These include protein C with its cofactor, protein S (A) and antithrombin (B) and tissue factor pathway inhibitor (C). Activated protein C/S inactivates factor Va and factor VIIIa. Antithrombin irreversibly binds to thrombin and factor Xa. Plasmin (D) breaks apart fibrin polymers to help dissolve the clot. Plasmin is activated from plasminogen by the action of plasminogen activators, including tissue plasminogen activator.

TF pathway inhibitor is the endogenous inhibitor for the factor Xa/factor Va complex.[12] It is secreted by activated platelets and found on the cell membranes of endothelial cells. Localization on endothelial surfaces may help reduce clot formation in areas of undamaged endothelium (see **Fig. 3**C).[15]

Fibrinolysis

Plasmin is the primary molecule that cleaves fibrin (see **Fig. 3**D). It is the active form of plasminogen. Plasminogen is processed into its active form by multiple types of plasminogen activators, the most potent of which is tissue plasminogen activator.[12,16] Plasminogen activators are released by endothelial cells because of a variety of stimuli, including the presence of thrombin. Fibrinolysis yields several different types of fibrin degradation products.[16]

Much more is known about the factors, proteins, cofactors, and cell surface molecules involved in the process of hemostasis, but a complete overview is beyond the scope of this article. Clearly, the process of maintaining hemostasis depends on complex interactions between systems that promote clot formation and systems that inhibit it. Disruption in this complex system can lead either to excessive bleeding or excessive and/or inappropriate clot formation.

BLEEDING DISORDERS

Excessive bleeding can result either from the reduced ability to form a clot or increased rate of dissolution of the clot. Disruption in clot formation can occur from multiple mechanisms (**Table 1**). First, decreased number of platelets can reduce clot formation. Disruption in the aggregation process of platelets can also slow the process. Bleeding can also result from issues with coagulation factors, either from lack of one or more factors or from the presence of an inhibitor, such as an autoantibody. Excessive activity from inhibitor molecules can reduce clot formation. Finally,

Table 1 Mechanisms of bleeding disorders	
Issues	**Examples**
1. Issues with platelets	
Decreased number caused by decreased production	Leukemia, lymphoma
Decreased number from increased destruction	Hypersplenism, autoantibodies
Decreased activation and aggregation	Nonsteroidal anti-inflammatory drugs, storage pool disorders
2. Issues with coagulation factors	
Genetic or acquired deficiency	Von Willebrand disease, hemophilia A, hemophilia B
Presence of an inhibitor	Factor VIII autoantibodies
3. Issues with fibrinolysis or inhibitors of coagulation	
Decreased activity of plasminogen inhibitors	Plasminogen activator inhibitor deficiency
4. Issues with blood vessel structure	Ehlers-Danlos syndrome, hereditary telangiectasias
5. Issues with other systems	Cushing disease Hypothyroidism Liver or kidney disease

overactive fibrinolysis mechanisms can result in bleeding as clots are dissolved before repair of the vessel wall is complete.[17–21]

Additionally, excessive bleeding can occur because of changes in blood vessel structure/integrity, such as connective tissue disorders, including Ehlers-Danlos syndrome, that cause spontaneous bleeding. Use of exogenous steroids or Cushing disease can also cause changes in the skin and vessels that lead to easier bruising/bleeding.[18,19]

Systemic illness, cancer, or nutritional deficiencies can also affect hemostasis. Hypothyroidism is associated with an increased risk of bleeding.[19,22] Vitamin K is a key component in the formation of factors II, VII, IX, and X, therefore poor nutrition can contribute to reduced levels of these factors.[18,19] The liver is responsible for the production of most of the proteins in the coagulation pathway with the exception of factor VIII. It is also responsible for production of thrombopoietin, which stimulates platelet production in the bone marrow. Therefore, impaired liver function can cause dysregulation of hemostasis by affecting platelet production and coagulation protein production.[18,19] Impaired renal function, especially in patients requiring dialysis, has been shown to cause dysregulation of hemostatic mechanisms. Patients on dialysis overall have a higher risk of bleeding and thrombosis compared with people without kidney disease.[23]

Finally, there are many drugs and supplements that alter the function and aggregation of platelets and reduce clotting.[19,21] Before an expensive and time-consuming diagnostic evaluation is undertaken, all possible contributing factors should be eliminated.

EVALUATION OF BLEEDING DISORDERS

A thorough history and physical examination is critical in the evaluation of bleeding disorders. Important information to elucidate includes details about prior bleeding episodes: spontaneous versus provoked; prolonged bleeding after surgery or dental procedures, including umbilical stump bleeding or circumcision; age of onset; associated symptoms; and sites of bleeding.[20–22] A complete list of medications, including all over-the-counter medications and supplements, is needed.[19,22] Also, a detailed family history is necessary to evaluate for inherited disorders. Answers to these questions can help guide testing. Mucocutaneous bleeding, such as nose bleeds, significant bleeding after dental procedures, or areas of bruising larger than ~ 5 cm, are more indicative of a platelet disorder, whereas bleeding into a joint or muscle, or delayed bleeding after surgery can indicate a coagulation cascade disorder.[19,21,22] A physical examination should include inspection of the skin for petechiae/purpura/ecchymoses and signs of liver disease; inspection of the mouth and gums for bleeding; and palpation for enlarged lymph nodes, liver, or spleen.[20,21]

INITIAL SCREENING TESTS
Complete Blood Count

A complete blood count (CBC) indicates issues with platelet count, including thrombocytopenia or thrombocytosis. It also can reveal anemia, which may be consistent with recurrent bleeding. An anemia panel may be indicated to confirm iron deficiency anemia from bleeding as opposed to other causes of anemia. It can also indicate the presence of a bone marrow disorder, such as leukemia, which can cause thrombocytopenia.[2,19–21]

Peripheral Blood Smear

Examination of a blood smear can assess for platelet morphology and red blood cell morphology. The presence of schistocytes, or red blood cell fragments, can indicate shearing from microangiopathic clot formation, such as with disseminated intravascular coagulation.[20,21]

Complete Metabolic Panel

A complete metabolic panel (CMP) can evaluate overall liver and kidney function.[21]

Prothrombin Time, Activated Partial Thromboplastin Time, Thrombin Time

Prothrombin time (PT) measures the activity of factors in the extrinsic and common pathways (factors VII, V, X, thrombin). For this assay, TF is added to plasma and the length of time to clot formation is measured in seconds. Any issue with factors in these pathways (either deficiency or inhibitor) delays formation of a clot, causing the PT to be longer than normal.[2,10,18]

Activated partial thromboplastin time (aPTT) measures the activity of factors in the intrinsic and common pathways (factors XII, XI, IX, VIII, V, X, thrombin). For this assay, a phospholipid mixture and a negatively charged surface are used to trigger activation of factor XII, leading to clot formation. Any issues with factors in these pathways (again either deficiency or inhibitor) delays clot formation, causing the aPTT to be longer than normal.[2,10,18]

Thrombin time (TT), also known as thrombin clotting time, is a measure of fibrinogen to fibrin conversion. In this assay, thrombin is added to plasma and the time is measured for clot formation. A delay in clot formation can indicate low levels of fibrinogen, decreased fibrin activity, or the presence of an inhibitor. Thrombin time is not available in all laboratories.[10,18]

These three measurements of clot formation help to identify issues with a subset of factors, helping to guide further testing (**Table 2**).[2,10,18,20–22]

FURTHER EVALUATION

Based on the initial laboratory studies and the patient's history and physical examination, further testing may be warranted to look for either a platelet disorder or a coagulation disorder. These tests are more specialized and expensive, so referral to a hematologist to guide further work-up is generally warranted.

Table 2
Interpretation of clotting assays

Test			Potential Coagulation Factors Affected	Other Possible Causes
PT	aPTT	TT		
Prolonged	Normal	Normal	Factor VII	
Normal	Prolonged	Normal	Factors VIII, IX, XI, XII	Lupus anticoagulant Von Willebrand disease
Prolonged	Prolonged	Normal	Factors II, V, X	Liver disease Vitamin K deficiency
Prolonged	Prolonged	Prolonged	Factor I (fibrinogen)	Liver disease
Normal	Normal	Normal	Factor XIII	Platelet dysfunction Excessive fibrinolysis Von Willebrand disease

Platelet Function and Platelet Aggregation Analysis

In years past, platelet function was measured using a bleeding time test in which a shallow cut was made on a patient's arm while a blood pressure cuff was applied at 40 mm Hg pressure. The length of time it took the cut to stop bleeding was related to platelet function, with decreased function causing longer bleeding times. However, this test is not routinely used in clinical laboratories.[2,10,22]

Platelet function analyzers, such as the PFA-100, are an alternative to the bleeding time test. In this test, blood is passed thru a membrane coated in collagen and either ADP or epinephrine. In normal blood, the platelets aggregate and occlude the membrane. This is called the "closure time." A prolonged closure time can indicate a platelet disorder. However, these analyzers are not sensitive enough for some of the more common platelet disorders.[2,10,21,22]

Platelet function is also measured using platelet aggregometry.[10,21] In platelet-rich plasma, the addition of an aggregation agonist causes the platelets to precipitate out of solution. This causes an increase in light transmission thru the container, which can be measured and plotted against time to yield an aggregation curve. In platelet aggregation studies, the patient's plasma is tested with various agonists and aggregation curves are compared with standardized samples.[10] Decreases in light transmission caused by reduced aggregation with a specific agonist are linked to a specific type of platelet disorder.[10]

Von Willebrand Factor

vWF is a key component involved in platelet binding to exposed collagen. Deficiencies in von Willebrand level or activity is the most common inherited disorder of hemostasis.[24] Laboratory assays are available to quantify the amount of vWF (antigen assays) and to evaluate its function (activity assays).[18,21,24] However, results of these assays are complicated because vWF is an acute phase reactant, and levels are increased because of inflammation/infection. vWF levels are also lower in people with type O blood.[24]

Coagulation Factor Assays

Once a potential issue is identified because of abnormal PT, aPTT, and/or TT tests, further evaluation helps narrow which factor is affected. The next step in evaluation is a mixing assay where the patient's plasma is mixed 1:1 with normal plasma then incubated. PT, aPTT, and/or TT tests are run on the mixed plasma at the beginning and at specific time intervals. If the issue is deficiency of a factor, then mixing with normal plasma will restore clotting ability and initially abnormal PT/aPTT/TT tests will now be within normal limits. If the issue is an inhibitor against a factor, then mixing with normal plasma will inhibit the factor in the normal plasma, therefore causing the initially abnormal PT/aPTT/TT tests to continue to be abnormally long for clot formation. In some cases, the initial test seems to be normal, but incubation causes further inhibition over time, so samples are incubated and tested at different time intervals (**Table 3**).[2,10,18,21,22]

If a deficiency in a factor is identified in the mixing assay, then the patient's plasma is mixed with different plasmas known to be deficient in a particular factor. For example, if the patient is deficient in factor IX, then mixing the patient's plasma with factor IX-deficient plasma leads to abnormal aPTT times. Mixing the patient's factor IX deficient plasma with plasma deficient in a different factor, however, rectifies the deficiency in each and therefore the clot formation times are normal.[2,10,25]

Table 3
Mixing studies

Sample	Initial	After (x) Time	Interpretation
1:1 mix patient plasma and normal plasma	Normal PT, aPTT, or TT	Normal PT, aPTT, or TT	Deficiency of a clotting factor
1:1 mix patient plasma and normal plasma	Normal or prolonged PT, aPTT, or TT	Prolonged PT, aPTT, or TT	Inhibitor against a clotting factor is present

Mixing studies are done after a patient's plasma has already had a prolonged PT, aPTT, or TT.

If an inhibitor to a factor is identified in the initial mixing assay, then the patient's plasma is tested for the presence of autoantibodies to each factor. The most common autoantibody inhibitor is against factor VIII.[10,26]

Factor XIII Assay

Factor XIIIa works to cross-link fibrin molecules to form a meshwork that stabilizes the clot. If there is a factor XIII deficiency or inhibitor, then a clot still forms but is not as stable. This means that the patient likely has normal PT, aPTT, TT tests and normal coagulation function assays. In this case, a clot solubility test can detect if the clot is less stable, indicating an issue with factor XIII.[20,25] Other assays can detect the level and functionality of factor XIII.[10,27]

Fibrinogen

Assays are available to measure the concentration of fibrinogen in blood (fibrinogen antigen test) and measure the activity of fibrinogen (thrombin time test).[10,25] Fibrinogen is an acute phase reactant, so levels are increased during infection and inflammation.[10]

CLOTTING DISORDERS

Inappropriate or excessive clot formation likewise has many causes. Structural variations can cause factors to be activated much easier, resulting in spontaneous clot formation. Also, variations that cause overproduction of one or more factors can result in excessive clot formation. Likewise, a deficiency in the activity of inhibitory molecules can promote clot formation. These deficiencies/inhibitors are either genetic or acquired.[28–30]

There are also many other causes to hypercoagulability that are not related to the hemostasis system.[28–30] These include

- Prolonged immobility: trauma, surgery, long car/plane trips, illness
- Cancer
- Pregnancy
- Slowed blood flow
  - Heart failure
  - Atrial fibrillation
  - Cirrhosis
- Changes in the endothelium
  - Vasculitis
  - Atherosclerosis
- Autoimmune disorders

Because there are so many possible causes for clot formation outside of the hemostasis system, laboratory evaluation is usually limited to those patients who have evidence of an unprovoked clot at an earlier age; recurrent clots; or a clot in an unusual area, such as mesenteric, renal, or hepatic vessels.[28,31] Additionally, if a patient has a clot, they may be on anticoagulant treatment. Therefore, it may be necessary to wait until treatment is completed before doing extensive laboratory evaluation, because many results are skewed in the presence of an anticoagulant.[2,28,31]

INITIAL TESTING
Complete Blood Count and Peripheral Blood Smear

Polycythemia and significant thrombocytosis can predispose to clot formation.[28]

Prothrombin Time, Activated Partial Thromboplastin Time

In general, PT and aPTT are likely normal. However, the process of clotting may be increased so that PT and/or aPTT are significantly shorter than normal. Also, the presence of a lupus anticoagulant (discussed later) causes aPTT to be longer than normal.[20,21,28]

Complete Metabolic Panel

A CMP can evaluate overall liver and kidney function.[28]

Fibrinogen

Fibrinogen is an acute phase reactant, and may remain elevated in the presence of chronic inflammation. Increased fibrinogen levels can predispose to clot formation.[28]

Protein C and Protein S, Antithrombin

Protein C and its cofactor, protein S, and antithrombin normally inhibit clot formation.[28,29] Assays are available to test the quantity of the protein (antigen assays) and the function of the protein (activity assays).[32]

Antiphospholipid Antibodies

Antiphospholipid antibodies are autoantibodies against phospholipid molecules in cell membranes. These can predispose to clot formation. They can develop in people with autoimmune diseases, such as lupus or rheumatoid arthritis, or can develop spontaneously. There are three main types: (1) lupus anticoagulants, (2) cardiolipin antibodies, and (3) β2 glycoprotein 1 antibodies.[2,28,33] Assays are available to test for the presence of each type.[28,33]

Homocysteine

Elevated levels of homocysteine are seen with vitamin B_{12} deficiency or nutritional deficiencies, or with genetic conditions, such as homocystinuria. Elevated levels had initially been associated with an increased risk of blood clot formation leading to an increased risk of stroke or heart attack. However, vitamin supplementation to correct deficiencies has not been shown to be effective at reducing homocysteine levels or reducing cardiovascular risks.[28,29] Additionally, newer studies showed that the risk was eliminated when adjusted for levels for factor VIII.[29] Therefore testing homocysteine levels has fallen out of favor.[29]

Factor V Leiden Mutation

Factor V Leiden mutation is the most common inherited cause of thrombophilia.[29] A mutation in the DNA causes a structural change that reduces the ability of protein

C to inactivate factor Va. This leads to increased levels of factor Va, which promotes clot formation.[28,29,32] Screening tests are available to screen for activated protein C resistance. If positive, then further DNA analysis is done to look for the mutation.[32]

Prothrombin 20210 Mutation

Prothrombin 20210 mutation is a change in the DNA that promotes increased synthesis of prothrombin. Increased levels of prothrombin in the blood promotes clot formation.[28,29,32] Testing is usually done with DNA analysis.[32]

D Dimer

Fibrin polymers are cleaved into fibrin degradation products of varying sizes. One such fibrin degradation product is called a D dimer. The level of D dimer products in the blood can be measured. This level is increased in the presence of increased clot formation, such as when there is a deep venous thrombosis or pulmonary embolism or disseminated intravascular coagulation.

MONITORING OF ANTICOAGULANTS

The past decade has seen a significant increase in the types of anticoagulants available. Some require frequent monitoring. Others do not need monitoring except in select situations. Tests available for monitoring are shown in **Table 4**.

Prothrombin Time, International Normalized Ratio

PT/international normalized ratio (INR) is largely used to monitor warfarin therapy.[2,34,35] Because of the variability in PT results between different laboratories, based on which specific assay reagents and machine were used, the INR was developed.[34,35] This is a laboratory-specific calculation that helps normalize PT results to an international standard based on specific machine and reagents. Therefore, the PT/INR results from one facility can be directly compared with PT/INR results from another facility. People on warfarin therapy therefore can have their level checked at different facilities without worrying about interlaboratory variability resulting in changes in their dosing levels.

Warfarin has been in use since the 1950s. It works by inhibiting an enzyme responsible for adding vitamin K cofactor to factors II, VII, IX, X, therefore those factors do not function normally.[34] Metabolism of warfarin is highly individual and affected by diet, therefore frequent monitoring is necessary to maintain a therapeutic level.[34,36]

Table 4 Anticoagulant monitoring		
Type of Drug	**Examples**	**Monitoring**
Vitamin K antagonist	Warfarin	PT/international normalized ratio
Activation of antithrombin	Unfractionated heparin	aPTT
Factor Xa inhibitors	Low-molecular-weight heparin (enoxaparin) Rivaroxaban Apixaban	Anti-Xa assays
Direct thrombin inhibitors	Argatroban Dabigatran	Thrombin time

PT/INR results are increased with some of the newer direct factor Xa inhibitors, such as rivaroxaban, when drug concentrations are higher than therapeutic levels. However, PT/INR results are increased even at therapeutic levels in some patients; in other patients, therapeutic levels do not increase the PT/INR. Therefore PT/INR is not used for monitoring the newer oral anticoagulants.[37]

Activated Partial Thromboplastin Time

aPTT is largely used to monitor unfractionated heparin levels, especially when given intravenously. Heparin works by binding to antithrombin and significantly increasing its binding to thrombin, therefore blunting clot formation. Heparin also binds to factor Xa and inactivates it.[34,35]

Anti-Xa Assays

Low molecular-weight-heparin, such as enoxaparin or fondaparinux, only bind to factor Xa.[34] Some of the newer oral anticoagulants are direct factor Xa inhibitors, including rivaroxaban and apixaban. Generally, these medications do not need monitoring.[34,35] However, in some situations, closer monitoring of drug levels may be needed to ensure therapeutic dosing. This includes significant obesity, renal impairment, or advanced age.[34,35] The anti-Xa assays indirectly measure the level of a factor Xa inhibitor. However, calibration curves must be developed at each laboratory for each type of factor Xa inhibitor, which limits the availability for monitoring these anticoagulants.[34,35,37]

Thrombin Time

Some of the newer anticoagulants are direct thrombin inhibitors, such as dabigatran and argatroban. Monitoring is done with TT measurements, but it is a qualitative test only.[34,35,37]

SUMMARY

The hemostasis system is a complex system designed to rapidly respond to damage to blood vessel integrity. However, changes in the quantity or functionality of any of the components can lead to excessive bleeding or excessive clotting. Evaluation of bleeding and clotting disorders begins with a thorough history and physical examination. Initial work-up for each type of disorder is similar: CBC, CMP, PT/INR, and aPTT. In assessment of bleeding disorders, a TT is also used. The CBC and CMP tests help to rule out causes unrelated to the hemostasis system and assess platelet quantity. PT/INR, aPTT, and TT help assess the components of the coagulation cascade. Based on these results, more specific tests are available to evaluate different components of the hemostasis system. For patients on anticoagulants, PT/INR, aPTT, or anti-Xa assays are used to monitor and maintain therapeutic levels.

REFERENCES

1. Fredenburgh JC, Weitz JI. Overview of hemostasis and thrombosis. In: Hoffman R, Benz EJ, Silberstein LE, et al, editors. Hematology: basic principles and practice. 7th edition. Philadelphia: Elsevier; 2018. p. 1831–42.
2. Konkle B. Bleeding and thrombosis. In: Longo DL, Fauci AS, Kasper DL, et al, editors. Harrison's principles of internal medicine. 18th edition. New York: McGraw-Hill; 2012. p. 457–64.
3. Kaushansky K. Megakaryopoiesis and thrombopoiesis. In: Kaushansky K, Lichtman MA, Prchal JT, et al, editors. Williams hematology, 9th edition. New York:

McGraw-Hill; Available at: http://accessmedicine.mhmedical.com.go.libproxy. wakehealth.edu/content.aspx?bookid=1581&sectionid=108078174. Accessed February 18, 2019.

4. Rand ML, Israels SJ. Molecular basis of platelet function. In: Hoffman R, Benz EJ, Silberstein LE, et al, editors. Hematology: basic principles and practice. 7th edition. Elsevier; 2018. p. 1870–84.

5. Giangrande PLF. Six characters in search of an author: the history of the nomenclature of coagulation factors. Br J Haematol 2003;121:703–12.

6. Brummel-Ziedins K, Mann KG. Molecular basis of blood coagulation. In: Hoffman R, Benz EJ, Silberstein LE, et al, editors. Hematology: basic principles and practice. 7th edition. Philadelphia: Elsevier; 2018. p. 1885–905.

7. Mann Kenneth G. Thrombin generation in hemorrhage control and vascular occlusion. Circulation 2011;124(2):225–35.

8. Goto S, Hasebe T, Takagi S. Platelets: small in size but essential in the regulation of vascular homeostasis – translation from basic science to clinical medicine. Circulation 2015;79:1871–81.

9. Mann KG, Brummel-Ziedins K, Orfeo T, et al. Models of blood coagulation. Blood Cells Mol Dis 2006;36(2):108–17.

10. Pai M. Laboratory evaluation of hemostatic and thrombotic disorders. In: Hoffman R, Benz EJ, Silberstein LE, et al, editors. Hematology: basic principles and practice. 7th edition. Philadelphia: Elsevier; 2018. p. 1922–31.

11. Bos MA, van 't Veer C, Reitsma PH. Molecular biology and biochemistry of the coagulation factors and pathways of hemostasis. In: Kaushansky K, Lichtman MA, Prchal JT, et al, editors. Williams hematology, 9th edition. New York: McGraw-Hill; Available at: http://accessmedicine.mhmedical.com.go.libproxy. wakehealth.edu/content.aspx?bookid=1581&sectionid=108079516. Accessed February 18, 2019.

12. Huntington JA, Baglin TP. Regulatory mechanisms in hemostasis. In: Hoffman R, Benz EJ, Silberstein LE, et al, editors. Hematology: basic principles and practice. 7th edition. Philadelphia: Elsevier; 2018. p. 1906–11.

13. Dahlbäck B, Villoutreix BO. Molecular recognition in the protein C anticoagulant pathway. J Thromb Haemost 2003;1:1525–34.

14. Bouwens EA, Stavenuiter F, Mosnier LO. Mechanisms of anticoagulant and cytoprotective actions of the protein C pathway. J Thromb Haemost 2013;11(Suppl 1): 242–53.

15. Wood JP, Ellery PE, Maroney SA, et al. Biology of tissue factor pathway inhibitor. Blood 2014;123(19):2934–43. Available at: https://doi.org/10.1182/blood-2013-11-512764.

16. Hajjar KA, Ruan J. Fibrinolysis and thrombolysis. In: Kaushansky K, Lichtman MA, Prchal JT, et al. editors. Williams hematology. 9th edition. New York: McGraw-Hill; Available at: http://accessmedicine.mhmedical.com.go.libproxy.wakehealth.edu/ content.aspx?bookid=1581&sectionid=108086006. Accessed February 17, 2019.

17. Bleeding disorders. American Society of Hematology. Available at: http://www. hematology.org/Patients/Bleeding.aspx. Accessed February 17, 2019.

18. Levi M, Seligsohn U, Kaushansky K. Classification, clinical manifestations, and evaluation of disorders of hemostasis. In: Kaushansky K, Lichtman MA, Prchal JT, et al. editors. Williams hematology. 9th edition. New York: McGraw-Hill; Available at: http://accessmedicine.mhmedical.com.go.libproxy.wakehealth.edu/content. aspx?bookid=1581&sectionid=108080936. Accessed February 17, 2019.

19. Hayward CPM. Clinical approach to the patient with bleeding or bruising. In: Hoffman R, Benz EJ, Silberstein LE, et al, editors. Hematology: basic principles and practice. 7th edition. Philadelphia: Elsevier; 2018. p. 1912–21.

20. Bashawri Layla AM, Ahmed Mirghani A. The approach to a patient with a bleeding disorder: for the primary care physician. J Family Community Med 2007;14(2):53–8.

21. Neutze D, Roque J. Clinical evaluation of bleeding and bruising in primary care. Am Fam Physician 2016;93(4):279–86.

22. Kruse-Jarres R, Singleton Tammuella C, Leissinger Cindy A. Identification and basic management of bleeding disorders in adults. J Am Board Fam Med 2014;27(4):549–64.

23. Lutz J, Menke J, Sollinger D, et al. Haemostasis in chronic kidney disease. Nephrol Dial Transplant 2014;29(1):29–40.

24. James P, Rydz N. Structure, biology, and genetics of von Willebrand Factor. In: Hoffman R, Benz EJ, Silberstein LE, et al, editors. Hematology: basic principles and practice. 7th edition. Philadelphia: Elsevier; 2018. p. 2051–63.

25. Peyvandi F, Menegatti M. Inherited deficiencies of coagulation factors II, V, V+VIII, VII, X, XI, and XIII. In: Kaushansky K, Lichtman MA, Prchal JT, et al. eds. Williams hematology. 9th edition. New York: McGraw-Hill; . Available at: http://accessmedicine.mhmedical.com.go.libproxy.wakehealth.edu/content.aspx?bookid=1581&sectionid=108083334. Accessed February 17, 2019.

26. Stowell SR, Lollar J, Meeks SL. Antibody-mediated coagulation factor deficiencies. In: Kaushansky K, Lichtman MA, Prchal JT, et al. eds. Williams hematology. 9th edition. New York: McGraw-Hill; . Available at: http://accessmedicine.mhmedical.com.go.libproxy.wakehealth.edu/content.aspx?bookid=1581&sectionid=108084072. Accessed February 17, 2019.

27. Nugent Diane J. Factor XIII deficiency laboratory evaluation. In: Rare coagulation disorders resource room. Available at: http://www.rarecoagulationdisorders.org/diseases/factor-xiii-deficiency/laboratory-evaluation. Accessed February 18, 2019.

28. Anderson JA, Hogg KE, Weitz JI. Hypercoagulable states. In: Hoffman R, Benz EJ, Silberstein LE, et al, editors. Hematology: basic principles and practice. 7th edition. Philadelphia: Elsevier; 2018. p. 2076–87.

29. Middeldorp S, Coppens M. Hereditary thrombophilia. In: Kaushansky K, Lichtman MA, Prchal JT, et al. eds. Williams hematology. 9th edition. New York: McGraw-Hill; Available at: http://accessmedicine.mhmedical.com.go.libproxy.wakehealth.edu/content.aspx?bookid=1581&sectionid=108084622. Accessed February 16, 2019.

30. Greaves M. Thrombophilia. Clin Med (Lond) 2001;1:432–5.

31. Stevens SM, Woller SC, Bauer KA, et al. Guidance for the evaluation and treatment of hereditary and acquired thrombophilia. J Thromb Thrombolysis 2016; 41(1):154–64.

32. Johnson NV, Khor B, Van Cott EM. Advances in laboratory testing for thrombophilia. Am J Hematol 2012;87:S108–12.

33. Rand JH, Wolgast L. The antiphospholipid syndrome. In: Kaushansky K, Lichtman MA, Prchal JT, et al. eds. Williams hematology. 9th edition. New York: McGraw-Hill; . Available at: http://accessmedicine.mhmedical.com.go.libproxy.wakehealth.edu/content.aspx?bookid=1581&sectionid=108084775. Accessed February 17, 2019.

34. Jaffer IH, Weitz JI. Antithrombotic drugs. In: Hoffman R, Benz EJ, Silberstein LE, et al, editors. Hematology: basic principles and practice. 7th edition. Philadelphia: Elsevier; 2018. p. 2168–88.
35. Harter K, Levine M, Henderson SO. Anticoagulation drug therapy: a review. West J Emerg Med 2015;16(1):11–7.
36. Verhoef TI, Redekop WK, Daly AK, et al. Pharmacogenetic-guided dosing of coumarin anticoagulants: algorithms for warfarin, acenocoumarol and phenprocoumon. Br J Clin Pharmacol 2014;77(4):626–41.
37. Samuelson BT, Cuker A. Measurement and reversal of the direct oral anticoagulants. Blood Rev 2016;31(1):77–84.

Diagnostics for White Blood Cell Abnormalities

Leukocytosis and Leukopenia

Jason Parente, MS, PA-C

KEYWORDS

- Leukocytosis • Leukopenia • Neutrophilia • Neutropenia • Diagnostic evaluation

KEY POINTS

- Define common terminology used in the evaluation of elevated or decreased white blood cell counts.
- Understand most common and most life-threatening etiologies of leukocytosis and leukopenia.
- Determine algorithmic approach to interpretation and management of abnormal white cell counts.

INTRODUCTION

The complete blood count (CBC) has become one of the most commonly ordered laboratory tests in clinical medicine today because it is readily available and provides a wealth of information. The caveat to its frequent use is that values often fall outside of a reference range presenting a diagnostic conundrum. Although subtle deviations are frequent, their presence can indicate a wide range of etiologies from benign outliers to the common cold or acute leukemia.[1] The substantial and seemingly endless amount of data obtained from CBCs can be overwhelming. This article provides common definitions and outlines diagnostic pathways to interpretation of leukocytosis and leukopenia within the CBC.

DEFINITIONS

"Leuko" originates from the Greek "leukos," meaning white. The medical suffixes "-cytosis" and "-philia" reference an increase in the number of cells, whereas "-penia" references a deficiency. "Leukocytosis" refers to white blood cell counts above the normal range. "Leukopenia" refers to white blood cell counts below the normal range.

Disclosure Statement: The author has no disclosures.
Physician Assistant Program, Northeastern University, 202 Robinson Hall, 360 Huntington Avenue, Boston, MA 02115, USA
E-mail address: J.parente@northeastern.edu

Physician Assist Clin 4 (2019) 625–635
https://doi.org/10.1016/j.cpha.2019.02.010
2405-7991/19/© 2019 Elsevier Inc. All rights reserved.

"Neutrophilia" refers to an elevated neutrophil count. "Neutropenia" refers to a neutrophil count below normal ranges. Leukocytosis elevation between 50,000 and 100,000/mm^3 is termed a leukemoid reaction. A myeloproliferative disorder is a disease of the bone marrow and blood that can create abnormal cells. Pancytopenia refers to decreased levels of all cell lines in the CBC.

COMPLETE BLOOD COUNT

The CBC assesses 3 major formed components—the red blood cells, the white blood cells, and the platelets.[2] In clinical practice, the white blood cell count is obtained as the primary marker of inflammation or infection and is a frequently used diagnostic tool. Therefore, it is important to understand the advantages, as well as limitations, of its use. Many disease processes are best described and understood by evaluating all components of the CBC in tandem.

All these elements develop from a common stem cell found in the bone marrow. More than 100 billion cells are produced every day in the adult human body through hematopoiesis within the bone marrow.[3] A majority of mature, and some immature cells, are found within the peripheral blood (**Fig. 1**).

LEUKOCYTOSIS AND NEUTROPHILIA

Leukocytosis refers to an elevated leukocyte count. Most assays define normal ranges for the white cell count as between 4500 and 11,000 cells/mm^3.[4] An elevated absolute neutrophil count (ANC) without a leukocytosis is referred to as "neutrophilia." When leukocytosis is combined with an elevated ANC, the term "neutrophilic leukocytosis" is used.[1] The distinctions in practice rarely have clinical implications. An elevated white blood cell count has many etiologies, including but not limited to infection, inflammatory processes, and malignancy, as well as normal variations including age, obesity, smoking, and pregnancy.[5] In the presence of leukocytosis, a peripheral smear may be helpful in determining an underlying etiology. The white cell lines evaluated in a peripheral

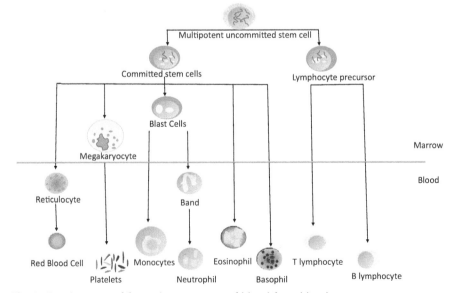

Fig. 1. Development of formed components of blood from blood marrow.

smear include monocytes, eosinophils, neutrophils, basophils and lymphocytes. **Table 1** lists reference ranges for differential white blood cell count. Leukocytosis exceeding 50,000 cells/mm^3 but less than 100,000 cells/mm^3 is referred to as a "leukemoid reaction" and may be seen in cases of severe infections including *Clostridium difficile*, tuberculosis, or sepsis.[6] Leukocytosis exceeding 100,000 cells/mm^3 is suggestive of a leukemia or myeloproliferative disorder and should raise suspicion for malignancy.

VARIATION

Multiple factors can affect normal white blood cell count ranges (**Table 2**). Two of the most common variations are younger age and pregnancy.[5] However, advanced age is not generally associated with elevated or decreased white blood cell counts in the absence of pathology and should not be used as a sole explanation for abnormal values.[7]

CAUSES OF LEUKOCYTOSIS AND NEUTROPHILIA

Approximately 30% to 60% of leukocytes are mature neutrophils. Neutrophils are produced and are largely present within the bone marrow. The entry of these cells into the circulation is regulated by multiple cytokines, and the peripheral white blood cell count is a transient reflection of neutrophils levels. Normally, they circulate for approximately 10 hours before entering tissues or undergoing cell death. Increased white blood cells in the periphery can be due to increased marrow production or demargination of peripheral blood neutrophils. Demargination refers to the process in which white cells are released from microcirculation or the vascular walls into the peripheral circulation.[8]

When evaluating neutrophilia, a left shift indicates the presence of immature neutrophils in the blood. The term is believed to have originated when cells were counted by hand with a manual machine. The most mature cells were accounted for with the right most button, and the immature forms known as bands, were counted with the leftmost button. Therefore, in the presence of a higher than normal number of immature neutrophils, there was a "left shift."[4] In clinically healthy patients, bands only compromise approximately 1% of neutrophils in the peripheral distribution.[9] A left shift is often mistakenly used to reference a neutrophil predominance, in which there is an increase in neutrophils, which may suggest a phase of an immune response, yet not the presence of immature forms.[8]

Infection

The most common cause of leukocytosis, usually neutrophilia, is secondary to infection.[7] Neutrophilia commonly occurs with bacterial infections. However, bacterial

Table 1		
Normal CBC differential ranges and percentages		
Cell Line	**Normal Cell Count (cells/mm^3)**	**Percentage of Total WBC**
Neutrophils	1830–7250	30%–60%
Lymphocytes	1500–4000	20%–50%
Monocytes	200–950	2%–10%
Eosinophils	0–700	0.3%–5%
Basophils	0–150	0.6%–1.8%

Data from Kasper DL, Fauci AS, Hauser SL, et al. Leukocytosis and leukopenia. In: Harrison's manual of medicine, 19e. New York: McGraw-Hill Education; 2016. Available at: accessmedicine. mhmedical.com/content.aspx?aid=1128783256. Accessed October 31, 2018.

Table 2
White blood cell count variation

Patient	Normal Leukocyte Count (cells/mm³)
Pregnant female in third trimester	5800–13,2000
Newborn infant	13,000–38,0000
Infant at 2 wk	5000–20,0000
Normal adult	4500–11,000

Data from Hoffman R, Benz EJ, Silberstein LE, et al, editors. Hematology: basic principles and practice. Philadelphia: Elsevier; 2018.

etiologies are not the only reason for elevated neutrophils. Neutrophilia may occur owing to viral infections, although its elevation is unpredictable.[7] A leukemoid reaction to most bacterial infections is uncommon, but if present should raise suspicion for severe infection.

Drug Induced

Steroids

Corticosteroids, which encompass glucocorticoids such as prednisone, are among the most common causes of drug-induced leukocytosis.[7] Steroids cause demargination of neutrophils from bone marrow stores into circulation and elevate peripheral cell counts. This transient elevation may be mistaken for infection.

Lithium

Lithium is often used for psychiatric illness and these patient populations may develop a leukocytosis without another contributing etiology. Lithium has been shown to stimulate neutrophil production through activation of colony stimulating factors.[5] Cell counts return to normal upon discontinuation of the medication.

Beta-adrenergic agonists

Beta agonists, such as albuterol and epinephrine, frequently stimulate the release of neutrophils from marginated storage pools and increase peripheral cell counts.[5]

Neoplasm

Sustained leukocytosis in the absence of other historical or physical examination findings should raise suspicion for neoplasm, especially if blast cells are present.[1,6,7] Hematologic malignancies can be associated with low, normal, or high white blood cell counts.[7] The 4 major subtypes of leukemia include acute lymphocytic leukemia, chronic myeloid leukemia, chronic lymphocytic leukemia, and acute myeloid leukemia.[10] Advanced age represents the largest population of these patients who also have the highest mortality.[7]

Smoking

Smoking has been associated with a mild elevation in white blood cell counts. White blood cell elevation can persist for up to 5 years after the cessation of smoking.[1,5]

Obesity

Obesity has been associated with a chronic, mild elevation in white blood cell counts.[6]

Splenectomy

Splenectomy is an important consideration in the evaluation of leukocytosis. After a splenectomy, patients may develop a mild, chronic leukocytosis. With time, the leukocytosis persists and becomes lymphocytic predominant.[6] Patients may have an exaggerated response to any of the aforementioned etiologies, resulting in a dramatic leukocytosis.

Stressful Stimuli

Leukocytosis can also occur in the setting of stress, exercise, seizure, or tissue necrosis (burn, shock, trauma, or infarction).[1,7]

ELEVATED CELL LINES

Evaluation of the peripheral blood smear can help determine conditions that typically elevate certain white blood cell lines (**Table 3**).

DIAGNOSTIC PATHWAY FOR LEUKOCYTOSIS

Fig. 2 presents a diagnostic pathway for leukocytosis.

Highlights of Leukocytosis

- Leukocytosis refers to an elevated leukocyte count.
- Leukocytosis and neutrophilia represent several different possible inflammatory responses, not just infection.
- Most assays define normal ranges for the white cell count as between 4500 and 11,000 cells/mm³.
- The 5 white cell lines evaluated in a peripheral smear are monocytes, eosinophils, neutrophils, basophils, and lymphocytes.
- Consider severe infection with leukocytosis from 50,000 to 100,000 cells/mm³.

Table 3
Conditions that elevate specific white blood cell lines

White Blood Cell Line	Abnormal Elevation	Conditions
Neutrophils	ANC >10,000 cells/mm³	Infection, drug induced, splenectomy, chronic inflammation, cigarette smoking, stress, exercise, malignancy, tissue necrosis, myeloproliferative disorders, hemolysis
Lymphocytes	Absolute lymphocyte count >5000 cells/mm³	Viral infections, bacterial infections (pertussis, bartonella, tuberculosis, syphilis, rickettsia, babesia), endocrine disorders, acute or chronic leukemia (chronic lymphocytic leukemia is the most common cause of lymphocyte count >10,000 cells/mm³)
Monocytes	Absolute monocyte count >800 cells/mm³	Infections (viral, fungal, tuberculosis, endocarditis, malaria, rickettsial disease), autoimmune disease (lupus, rheumatoid arthritis, giant cell arteritis, inflammatory bowel disease)
Eosinophils	Absolute eosinophil count >500 cells/mm³	Parasitic infection, allergic disease, drug induced, dermatologic, collagen vascular diseases, neoplasm
Basophils	Absolute basophil count >100 cells/mm³	Allergic conditions, leukemias, chronic inflammatory disorders

Data from Kasper DL, Fauci AS, Hauser SL, et al. Leukocytosis and leukopenia. In: Harrison's manual of medicine, 19e. New York: McGraw-Hill Education; 2016. Available at: accessmedicine. mhmedical.com/content.aspx?aid=1128783256. Accessed October 31, 2018.

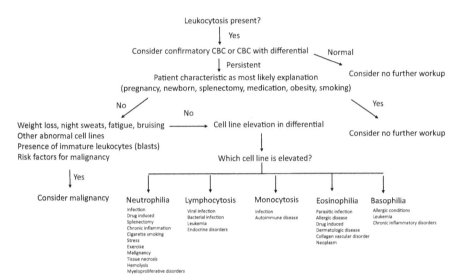

Fig. 2. Diagnostic pathway for leukocytosis.

- Consider malignancy or myelodysplastic syndrome with leukocytosis of greater than 100,000 cells/mm³
- Consider patient characteristics when evaluating leukocytosis.

LEUKOPENIA AND NEUTROPENIA

Leukopenia refers to a total leukocyte count less than 4500 cells/mm³ in most assays.[6] Neutropenia refers to an ANC of less than 2000 cells/mm³. The degree of neutropenia may be classified as mild (ANC 1000–2000 cells/mm³), moderate (ANC 500–1000 cells/mm³), or severe (ANC <500 cells/mm³)[1] (**Table 4**).

The pathophysiology of decreased neutrophils is the result of increased destruction or decreased production.[6] Patients with neutropenia are increasingly susceptible to bacterial and fungal infections.[11] Therefore, it is important to determine the degree of neutropenia, the chronicity of neutropenia, and any associated infectious symptoms. The risk of infection is inversely related to the degree of neutropenia, where severe neutropenia carries the greatest risk.[8] In the presence of fever and neutropenia, patients typically require early, broad-spectrum intravenous antibiotics, even before the source can be identified.

Table 4 Degree of neutropenia	
Degree	**ANC cells/mm³**
Normal neutrophil counts	>2000
Mild neutropenia	1000–2000
Moderate neutropenia	500–1000
Severe neutropenia	<500

Data from Brar RS, Schrier SL. Consultative hematology. In: Kaushansky K, Lichtman MA, Prchal JT, et al, editors. Williams hematology, 9e. New York: McGraw-Hill Education; 2015. Available at: accessmedicine.mhmedical.com/content.aspx?aid=1121088548. Accessed October 31, 2018.

CAUSES OF LEUKOPENIA AND NEUTROPENIA

Leukopenia, which is most commonly the result of neutropenia, can be either acquired or congenital. Acquired neutropenia can be the result of medications, infections, nutritional deficiency, hematologic disease, and autoimmune disease (**Box 1**).

Drug Induced

Drug-induced neutropenia is the most common cause of neutropenia.[12] Chemotherapy agents are the most common drugs which induce neutropenia. Other drugs include antibiotics, antiepileptic medication, immunosuppressant medication, and alcohol (**Box 2**).

Infection

Both viral and bacterial infectious agents may cause leukopenia. Viral infections include influenza, hepatitis, human immunodeficiency virus, Epstein–Barr virus, measles, varicella, parvovirus, and cytomegalovirus. Atypical infections including malaria, typhoid fever, tuberculosis, ehrlichiosis, and some staphylococcal infections are also associated with neutropenia.[12] Perhaps the most significant consideration of neutropenia is that its presence may indicate sepsis, which is also known to cause a significant leukocytosis.[6,12] Fevers in neutropenia should always be presumed to be infectious until proven otherwise and there should be a low threshold to initiate broad-spectrum intravenous antibiotics and determine the source.[11]

Nutritional Deficiency

Several vitamin and mineral deficiencies, including B_{12}, folate, and copper, have been associated with neutropenia.

Hematologic Disease

Leukemia, aplastic anemia, and myelodysplastic syndromes are associated with neutropenia.[12]

Autoimmune Disease

Neutropenia can also be the result of autoimmune disease, both primary and secondary. Rheumatoid arthritis, systemic lupus erythematosus, Wegener granulomatosis, and hyperthyroid have been associated with neutropenia.[12] In systemic lupus erythematosus, nearly one-half of patients are neutropenic.[1]

Box 1
Differential diagnosis of acquired neutropenia

Infection

After infection

Drug induced

Immune neutropenia

Bone marrow failure

Hypersplenism

Nutritional deficiency

Data from Berliner, N. Leukocytosis and leukopenia. In: Russell LF, Goldman L, Schafer AI, editors. Goldman's Cecil medicine. Philadelphia: Elsevier; 2016.

Box 2
Drugs associated with neutropenia

Antibiotics: vancomycin, penicillins, sulfa, linezolid, chloramphenicol

Antithyroid medications: methimazole and propylthiouracil

Cardiovascular: ticlopidine, procainamide

Antipsychotics: clozapine, olanzapine, chlorpromazine

Anticonvulsants: phenytoin, carbamazepine, valproic acid

Anti-inflammatory: indomethacin, sulfasalazine, phenylbutazone

H2 blockers: cimetidine, ranitidine

Analgesics: dipyrone

Antineoplastic: rituximab

Anthelmintic: levamisole

Data from Brar RS, Schrier SL. Consultative hematology. In: Kaushansky K, Lichtman MA, Prchal JT, et al, editors. Williams hematology, 9e. New York: McGraw-Hill Education; 2015. Available at: accessmedicine.mhmedical.com/content.aspx?aid=1121088548. Accessed October 31, 2018.

Congenital

There are several genetic predispositions that result in chronically low neutrophil counts. These conditions exist as a primary neutrophil disorder, as seen with benign familial neutropenia or severe congenital neutropenia, but also may be the result of other congenital syndromes that are associated with neutropenia. Patients with chronic or congenital neutropenia syndromes experience infection at much lower rates than those with acquired neutropenia, as seen in chemotherapy[12] (**Box 3**).

Depressed Cell Lines

Evaluating the differential smear can help to identify underlying etiologies. Although used less frequently in clinical practice than the differential of leukocytosis, specific

---

Box 3
Differential diagnosis of congenital neutropenia

Benign familial neutropenia

Severe congenital neutropenia

Cyclic neutropenia

Dyskeratosis congenita

Fanconi anemia

Chediak–Higashi syndrome

Shwachmann–Diamond syndrome

Griscelli syndrome type II

Hermansky–Pudlak syndrome

Glycogen storage disease

Data from Berliner, N. Leukocytosis and leukopenia. In: Russell LF, Goldman L, Schafer AI, editors. Goldman's Cecil medicine. Philadelphia: Elsevier; 2016.

cell lines may see a decrease in absolute cell counts. The most common causes include acute stressful reactions and glucocorticoid therapy[6] (**Table 5**).

DIAGNOSTIC PATHWAY FOR LEUKOPENIA

Fig. 3 presents a diagnostic pathway for leukopenia.

Highlights of Leukopenia

- Leukopenia refers to a decreased leukocyte count of less than 4500 cells/mm^3.
- Leukopenia can be either congenital or acquired.
- Neutropenia is associated with an increased risk of infection.
- The acuity and degree of neutropenia can help to determine the etiology and risk of infection.

PRACTICE QUESTIONS

Question 1

Neutrophilia is always secondary to a bacterial infection.
  True
  False

Question 2

A 47-year-old man is found to have leukocytosis. The provider is concerned about a parasitic infection. Which differential within the white blood cell count is *most likely* to be elevated?
A. Basophils
B. Eosinophils
C. Lymphocytes
D. Monocytes
E. Neutrophils

Table 5
Conditions that depress certain white blood cell lines

White Blood Cell Line	Abnormal Range	Conditions
Neutrophils	ANC <2000 cells/mm^3	Medication, severe bacterial infection, viral infection, sepsis, nutritional deficiency, hematologic disease, autoimmune disease, congenital disorders
Lymphocytes	Absolute lymphocyte count <1000 cells/mm^3	Acute stressful illness, HIV, immunosuppressants (steroids, alcohol), bone marrow failure
Monocytes	Absolute monocyte count <100 cells/mm^3	Acute stressful illness, glucocorticoid therapy, aplastic anemia, leukemia (hairy cell leukemia), chemotherapy
Eosinophils	Absolute eosinophil count <50 cells/mm^3	Acute stressful illness, glucocorticoid therapy, HIV

Abbreviation: HIV, human immunodeficiency virus.
  Data from Kasper DL, Fauci AS, Hauser SL, et al. Leukocytosis and leukopenia. In: Harrison's manual of medicine, 19e. New York: McGraw-Hill Education; 2016. Available at: accessmedicine. mhmedical.com/content.aspx?aid=1128783256. Accessed October 31, 2018; and Brar RS, Schrier SL. Consultative hematology. In: Kaushansky K, Lichtman MA, Prchal JT, et al, editors. Williams Hematology, 9e. New York: McGraw-Hill Education; 2015. Available at: accessmedicine.mhmedical. com/content.aspx?aid=1121088548. Accessed October 31, 2018.

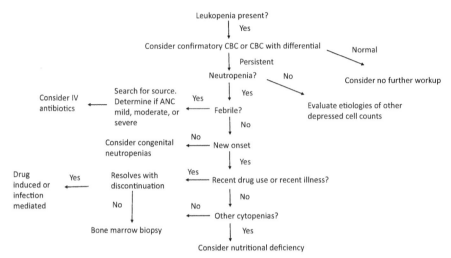

Fig. 3. Diagnostic pathway for leukopenia.

Question 3

A 60-year-old woman with a history of breast cancer currently undergoing chemotherapy presents for evaluation of fever. After obtaining a complete cell count with differential it is determined she has evidence of severe neutropenia. Which of the following ANCs correlates with this finding?

A. Greater than 2000 cell/mm^3
B. Between 1000 and 2000 cell/mm^3
C. Between 500 and 1000 cell/mm^3
D. Less than 500 cell/mm^3

Question 4

A 14-year-old boy is evaluated for fever and sore throat. He has no prior surgeries and takes no medications. A complete blood cell count reveals leukocytosis with an elevated lymphocyte count. What is the most likely etiology?

A. Bacterial infection
B. Parasitic infection
C. Malignancy
D. Splenectomy
E. Viral infection

REFERENCES

1. Brar RS, Schrier SL. Consultative hematology. In: Kaushansky K, Lichtman MA, Prchal JT, et al, editors. Williams hematology, 9e. New York: McGraw-Hill Education; 2015. Available at: accessmedicine.mhmedical.com/content.aspx?aid=1121088548. Accessed October 31, 2018.

2. Aster JC. Introduction to blood and hematopoietic tissues. In: Aster JC, Bunn HF, editors. Pathophysiology of blood disorders, 2e. New York: McGraw-Hill Education; 2016. Available at: accessmedicine.mhmedical.com/content.aspx?aid=1133369477. Accessed October 31, 2018.

3. Davoren JB, Wang S. Blood disorders. In: Hammer GD, McPhee SJ, editors. Pathophysiology of disease: an introduction to clinical medicine, 7e. New York:

McGraw-Hill Education; 2013. Available at: accessmedicine.mhmedical.com/content.aspx?aid=1100858295. Accessed November 4, 2018.

4. Gomella LG, Haist SA. Laboratory diagnosis: clinical hematology. In: Clinician's pocket reference: the Scut monkey, 11e. . New York: The McGraw-Hill Companies; 2007 [Chapter 5]. Available at: accessmedicine.mhmedical.com/content.aspx?aid=2700348. Accessed November 4, 2018.

5. Hoffman R, Benz EJ, Silberstein LE, et al. Hematology: basic principles and practice. In: Hematology. 6e. Philadelphia: Elsevier; 2018.

6. Kasper DL, Fauci AS, Hauser SL, et al. Leukocytosis and leukopenia. In: Harrison's manual of medicine, 19e. New York: McGraw-Hill Education; 2016. Available at: accessmedicine.mhmedical.com/content.aspx?aid=1128783256. Accessed October 31, 2018.

7. Klepin HD, Powell BL. White cell disorders. In: Halter JB, Ouslander JG, Studenski S, et al, editors. Hazzard's geriatric medicine and gerontology, 7e. New York: McGraw-Hill Education; 2017. Available at: accessmedicine.mhmedical.com/content.aspx?aid=1136596442. Accessed October 31, 2018.

8. Dale DC, Welte K. Neutropenia and neutrophilia. In: Kaushansky K, Lichtman MA, Prchal JT, et al, editors. Williams hematology, 9e. New York: McGraw-Hill Education; 2015. Available at: accessmedicine.mhmedical.com/content.aspx?aid=1121095938. Accessed October 31, 2018.

9. Lichtman M, Shafer J, Felgar R, et al. Neutrophils, non-clonal abnormalities. In: Lichtman's atlas of hematology 2016. New York: McGraw-Hill Education; 2017. Available at: accessmedicine.mhmedical.com/content.aspx?aid=1138037206. Accessed January 14, 2019.

10. Kemp WL, Burns DK, Brown TG. Hematopathology. In: Pathology: the big picture. New York: The McGraw-Hill Companies; 2008 [Chapter 12]. Available at: accessmedicine.mhmedical.com/content.aspx?aid=57052907. Accessed January 14, 2019.

11. Damon LE, Babis Andreadis C. Blood disorders. In: Papadakis MA, McPhee SJ, Rabow MW, editors. Current medical diagnosis & treatment 2019. New York: McGraw-Hill Education; 2019. Available at: accessmedicine.mhmedical.com/content.aspx?aid=1154896061. Accessed October 31, 2018.

12. Berliner N. Chapter 170: Leukocytosis and Leukopenia. In: Cecil RL, Russell LF, et al, editors. Goldman's Cecil medicine. 24e. Philadelphia, PA: Elsevier/Saunders; 2012.

Complete Blood Cell Count Interpretation for Hypoproliferative Anemias

Dipu Patel, MPAS, PA-C

KEYWORDS

- Complete blood count • Anemia • Red blood cells • Iron deficiency • Thalassemia
- Folate deficiency • B12 deficiency • Chronic disease

KEY POINTS

- The complete blood cell count (CBC) is one of the most commonly ordered blood tests.
- The CBC provides insight into several disease processes as well as normal hematopoietic physiology.
- Interpretation of the CBC is a skill that every provider must have facility with.
- A CBC provides insight into various disease processes and pathologies and, based on patient history, can be a valuable tool in diagnosing anemia.

INTRODUCTION

The complete blood cell count (CBC) is one of the most commonly ordered blood tests. It provides insight into several disease processes as well as normal hematopoietic physiology. Values of erythrocytes, leukocytes, and thrombocytes are included in the basic panel. This article discusses the interpretation of erythrocytes, or red blood cells (RBCs), in the context of diagnosing various types of anemia.

The average life span of an average RBC is 100 days to 120 days.[1] The mean corpuscular volume (MCV), mean corpuscular hemoglobin (MCH) concentration, and MCH are collectively known as the red cell indices. Of the 3 values, MCV is used to further delineate anemias into 3 broad categories of normocytic, microcytic, and macrocytic types. Normocytic anemias have MCV values of 80 fL and 100 fL; microcytic anemias have MCV values of less than 80 fL; and macrocytic anemias have MCV values greater than 100 fL.[2] Additionally, red cell distribution width (RDW) is helpful. The RDW is a measure of the size distribution and volume of a red cell. It aids in distinguishing anemias; for example, RDW is elevated in iron deficiency

Disclosure Statement: None.
Northeastern University, Bouve College of Health Sciences, Physician Assistant Program, 360 Huntington Avenue, R202, Boston, MA 02155, USA
E-mail address: d.pateljunankar@neu.edu

Physician Assist Clin 4 (2019) 637–647
https://doi.org/10.1016/j.cpha.2019.02.011
2405-7991/19/© 2019 Elsevier Inc. All rights reserved.

anemia and sometimes in megaloblastic anemias but does not change in anemia of chronic disease (ACD).[3] **Table 1** provides an overview of the anemias discussed in this article.

IRON METABOLISM AND STORAGE

Iron metabolism and storage have an impact on several organs. Disease in any of the organs affected by iron metabolism can lead to various signs and symptoms of anemia. **Fig. 1** demonstrates typical absorption and distribution for storage. After absorption of iron from dietary intake via the intestinal villi, transferrin transports iron to the marrow for production of RBCs, to the liver for storage and recycling, and to the muscles for the production of myoglobin. On average, 1 mL of red cells contains 1 mg of iron.[1] Iron is stored in the form of ferritin in various organs, such as the spleen, marrow, and skeletal muscle.

To maintain a balance of supply and demand, hepcidin inhibits iron transportation when high levels of iron are present. Hepcidin aids in decreasing absorption, decreasing recycling, and decreasing storage of iron.[4–7]

CLASSIFICATION OF ANEMIAS

Anemias may be classified in several ways. The most common methodology is physiologically. Broadly speaking, anemias can be hypoproliferative or hyperproliferative. **Fig. 2** outlines algorithmically the anemias discussed in this article. This physiologic classification is based on the reticulocyte index. Reticulocytes are the precursors to mature RBCs and, therefore, offer insight into the state of the bone marrow. A low reticulocyte count indicates inadequate red cell production whereas a high reticulocyte count indicates increased red cell production, which points to increased red cell destruction. The reticulocyte index is calculated using the reticulocyte count, multiplying it by a patient's hematocrit, and dividing by 40 for women or by 45 for men (average baseline hematocrit).

Hypoproliferative anemias usually are a result of inadequate production of RBCs by the marrow. Inadequate production may be due to several factors, such as lacking appropriate ingredients for the production of RBCs (iron, vitamin B12, and folate) or from marrow dysfunction due to iatrogenic reasons. On the other hand, hyperproliferative anemias are a result of increased destruction and/or loss of RBCs, in which the bone marrow is unable to appropriately compensate for the losses.

Microcytic Anemia (Mean Corpuscular Volume Less Than 80 fL)

Microcytic anemias are by far the most common of all the anemias. Of the two discussed in this article, iron deficiency anemia by far is the most common, affecting women of childbearing age, patients with gastrointestinal issues, and women with a history of menometrorrhagia.[8]

Serum ferritin, serum iron, and total iron binding capacity (TIBC) measure iron supply.[1]

Table 1 Hypoproliferative anemias		
Microcytic	**Normocytic**	**Macrocytic**
Iron deficiency	ACD	Vitamin B_{12} deficiency
Thalassemias		Folic acid deficiency

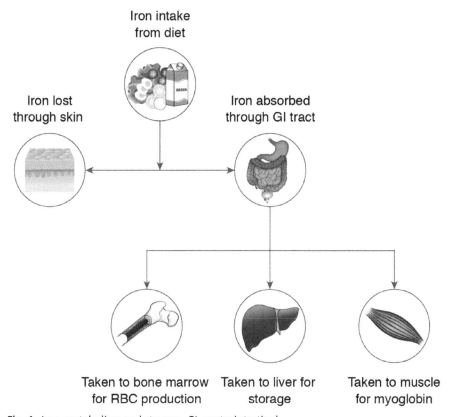

Fig. 1. Iron metabolism and storage. GI, gastrointestinal.

Serum ferritin is an indication of iron stores and is decreased in iron deficiency anemia.

TIBC is a measure of the availability of iron binding sites on transferrin.[6] TIBC aids in diagnosing both iron deficiency and iron overload diseases, such as hemochromatosis. In iron deficiency anemia, TIBC increases as the body attempts to maximize utilization of iron stores.[9]

Transferrin saturation, represented as a percentage, is calculated by dividing the serum iron by the TIBC and multiplying by 100. Transferrin saturations of less than 20% indicate iron deficiency anemia.[10]

Iron deficiency anemia typically is due to 1 of 3 reasons: decreased absorption, increased requirement, and blood loss. Examples of decreased absorption include gastric bypass surgery, celiac sprue, and other factors that have an impact on normal absorption of iron from dietary intake. Increased requirement typically is due to pregnancy. Finally, blood loss may be due to menstruation, gastrointestinal loss, or donation of blood. Presentation of iron deficiency anemia can range from asymptomatic to weakness, fatigue, shortness of breath, dizziness, headaches, and pica. Physical examination may reveal tachycardia, generalized pallor, and pale conjunctiva. Glossitis, koilonychia, and esophageal webbing are rare findings associated with iron deficiency anemia, and should prompt further work-up for other systemic conditions.

Diagnosis of iron deficiency anemia is initiated by a suspicion of the diagnosis based on history and physical examination, then by performing a CBC, specifically

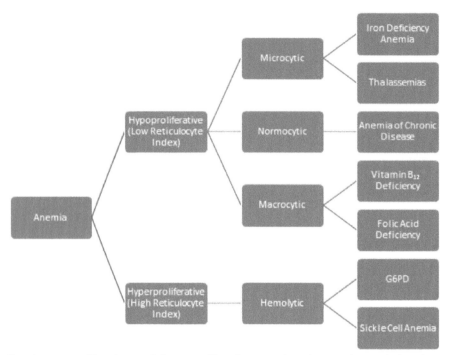

Fig. 2. Hypoproliferative and hyperproliferative anemias. G6PD, glucose-6-phosphate dehydrogenase.

interpreting the hemoglobin, RDW, MCV, and iron studies, including serum iron, serum ferritin, and TIBC, as seen in **Table 2**. RBCs on a peripheral smear appear microcytic and hypochromic (**Figs. 3** and **4**).

Thalassemia is an inherited disorder of hemoglobin synthesis. The disorder decreases production of globin chains, thereby leading to a microcytic anemia. It is categorized into α-thalassemia and β-thalassemia, depending on which chain is affected. α-Thalassemia is primarily due to gene deletions, leading to reduced α-globin chain synthesis, whereas β-thalassemia is typically caused by point mutations.

α-Thalassemia is more commonly seen in patients with Southeast Asian and Chinese descent. The patient without thalassemia has 4 copies of α-globin chains, 1 pair from each parent. If a patient has 3 copies, the patient is considered a silent carrier; if a patient has 2 copies, the patient has α-thalassemia trait (also known as α-thalassemia minor); if a patient has 1 copy of α-globin chain, it is known as hemoglobin H

Table 2
Iron studies in microcytic, hypochromic anemias

	Microcytic, Hypochromic	
Iron Studies	Iron Deficiency Anemia	Thalassemia
Serum ferritin	Low	Normal or increased
Serum iron	Low	Normal or increased
TIBC	Increased	Normal or increased
Transferrin saturation	Low	Normal or increased

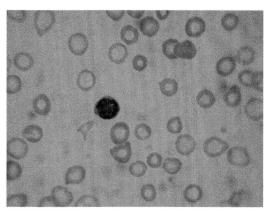

Fig. 3. Microcytic, hypochromic RBCs with anisocytosis. (Note: normal RBCs are approximately the size of the nucleus of a lymphocyte.) Wright's stain, original magnification 1000×. (*Courtesy of* James A. Van Rhee, MS, PA-C and Jane McDaniel, MS, MLS, SC.)

(HbH) disease (also known as α-thalassemia intermedia); and, lastly, if a patient has no copies of α-globin, it is known as Hemoglobin Barts or Hb Barts or hydrops fetalis syndrome and results in death in utero. **Table 3** provides a description of α-thalassemia genotypes.

α-Thalassemia patients may present with generalized symptoms, such as fatigue, weakness, and pallor; to more marked symptoms and signs, such as splenomegaly, skin ulcers, fever, and jaundice; or may be asymptomatic if they are silent carriers or have α-thalassemia trait. Diagnostic work-up shows a normocytic anemia progressing over time to a microcytic, hypochromic anemia, with normal reticulocyte counts for silent carriers and α-thalassemia trait. For α-thalassemia intermedia, reticulocytosis is noted due to increased hemolysis, and target cells (**Fig. 5**) and Heinz bodies re noted on peripheral smear. Ferritin level should be ordered to rule out iron deficiency anemia. Hemoglobin electrophoresis is the diagnostic study of choice. α-Thalassemia carrier and trait do not require active treatment but should be transfused as needed. Those with HbH disease require transfusions for hemoglobin levels less than 7 g/dL.[11]

β-Thalassemia is primarily seen in patients of Mediterranean descent, such as patients of Italian and Greek descent. Because β-thalassemia is caused by mutations,

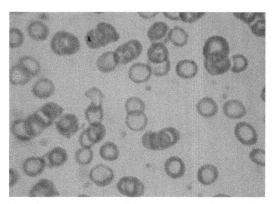

Fig. 4. Microcytic, hypochromic RBCs. Wright's stain, original magnification 1000×. (*Courtesy of* James A. Van Rhee, MS, PA-C and Jane McDaniel, MS, MLS, SC.)

Table 3
α-Thalassemia genotypes

No. of Alpha Chains	Name	Genotype	Anemia	Symptoms
4	Normal	αα/αα	None	None
3	Carrier	αα and α-	None	Make enough hemoglobin, no symptoms
2	Trait/minor	αα/- or α-/α-	Mild	Mild symptoms
1	HbH disease	α-/-	Moderate	Ischemia, target cells, Heinz bodies
0	Hydrops fetalis	-/-	Fatal	Fatality

it is classified as major (homozygous) or minor (heterozygous). In β-thalassemia major, there is severely limited production of β-globin due to the mutation. In β-thalassemia minor (also known as β-thalassemia trait), there is reduced β-globin chain production. **Box 1** and **Table 4** list the β-thalassemia alleles and genotypes.

Patients with β-thalassemia minor or trait are asymptomatic, whereas those with β-thalassemia major present similarly to α-thalassemia intermedia, with pallor, irritability, hepatosplenomegaly, and target cells apparent on peripheral smear (see **Fig. 5**). Diagnostic work-up is similar to α-thalassemia. Iron deficiency anemia should be ruled out with a ferritin level. Patients with β-thalassemia minor typically do not require treatment other than supportive measures, such as blood transfusions, as needed. β-Thalassemia major patients, however, may require regular blood transfusions, folic acid supplementation, and splenectomy, depending on the severity of symptoms.[12]

Normocytic Anemia (Mean Corpuscular Volume 80–100 fL)

Normocytic anemias are classified further into hemolytic or nonhemolytic. Hemolytic anemia includes both acquired and congenital forms (See James A. Van Rhee's article, "Hemolytic Anemia: Mass Destruction," in this issue). ACD is a form of nonhemolytic, normocytic anemia. ACD often is used interchangeably with anemia of chronic disorder or anemia of chronic inflammation. It often is seen in patients with

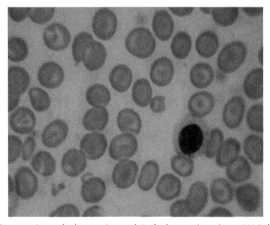

Fig. 5. Target cells seen in α-thalassemia and β-thalassemia minor. Wright's stain, original magnification 1000×. (*Courtesy of* James A. Van Rhee, MS, PA-C and Jane McDaniel, MS, MLS, SC.)

Box 1	
β-Thalassemia alleles	
Allele	**Genotype**
No mutation	β
Mutation leads to formation of no beta chains	β0
Mutation allows formation of some beta chains	β+

chronic kidney disease, malignancies, and various infectious and inflammatory disorders. The presentation of ACD is similar to other anemias and symptoms typically are a reflection of a decrease of RBC production by the bone marrow. Signs and symptoms of ACD vary depending on the underlying condition; therefore, providers should assess both for underlying etiology as well as have a higher degree of suspicion for ACD in the setting of certain chronic diseases. **Table 5**[13,14] provides a brief list of conditions associated with ACD.

The hallmark of ACD is a decrease in serum iron.[13,14] Additionally, transferrin levels are low, and saturation of transferrin is normal to low. Serum ferritin levels are normal or increased. Elevated serum ferritin levels should take into account underlying inflammatory conditions, because ferritin is an acute-phase reactant and may be elevated in malignancy and autoimmune diseases. Treatment of ACD should be focused on treating the underlying condition. Consideration also should be given to initiation of erythropoietin in those patients who are symptomatic or whose treatment may worsen anemia.

Macrocytic Anemia (Mean Corpuscular Volume Greater Than 100 fL)

Macrocytic anemias, also collectively known as megaloblastic anemias, are named as such due to the red cell morphology seen on peripheral smear. They include vitamin B_{12} (cobalamin) deficiency and folic acid deficiency anemias. The frequency of megaloblastic anemias tends to be higher in countries where malnutrition is common.[15,16] Vitamin B_{12}, a water-soluble vitamin, is found in meat, dairy, and fish, typically foods of animal origin. In contrast, folate is found in leafy greens and nuts. Both cobalamin and folate are necessary for DNA synthesis of dividing cells.[15]

The typical patient presenting with vitamin B_{12} deficiency may provide a history of gastrectomy, follow a strict vegetarian diet, or have a history of disorders that affect the terminal ileum (where vitamin B_{12} is absorbed), such as inflammatory bowel disease. In addition to the typical signs and symptoms of anemia (tachycardia, dyspnea, and fatigue), patients with vitamin B_{12} deficiency may present with glossitis, hyperpigmentation of skin, and peripheral neuropathy. There can be many overlapping signs and symptoms between vitamin B_{12} deficiency and folic acid deficiency; therefore, work-up for both should be initiated simultaneously. Initial work-up should include

Table 4				
β-Thalassemia genotypes				
Mutation	**Name**	**Genotype**	**Anemia**	**Symptoms**
Normal production	Normal	β	None	None
Some beta chains are formed	Minor	β+/β β0/β	Mild	Mild symptoms of anemia
Some beta chains are formed	Intermedia	β+/β+ β0/β+	Moderate	Normal life, occasional transfusions
No beta chains are formed	Major	β0/β0	Severe	Splenomegaly, bone deformities, death by 20

Table 5	
Diseases associated with anemia of chronic disease	
Category	**Diseases Associated with Anemia of Chronic Disease**
Infection	AIDS/HIV, tuberculosis, malaria (contributory), osteomyelitis, chronic abscesses, sepsis
Inflammation	Rheumatoid arthritis, other rheumatologic disorders, inflammatory bowel diseases, systemic inflammatory response syndrome
Malignancy	Carcinomas, multiple myeloma, lymphomas
Cytokine dysregulation	Anemia of aging

CBC, red cell indices, reticulocyte count, serum vitamin B_{12} levels, serum folate levels, serum methylmalonic acid (MMA) levels, and serum homocysteine levels. In addition, lactate dehydrogenase levels re elevated. In the typical megaloblastic picture, neutrophils appear hypersegmented and red cells appear large (**Figs. 6** and **7**).

MMA is an important factor in red cell metabolism.[1] Both homocysteine and MMA levels are elevated in vitamin B_{12} deficiency. In folic acid deficiency, homocysteine levels are elevated but MMA levels are not. This helps differentiate vitamin B_{12} deficiency from folic acid deficiency.

Treatment of vitamin B_{12} deficiency typically includes 1000 µg of intramuscular vitamin B_{12} daily, followed by weekly dosing until the hematocrit is within normal range.[15] More aggressive treatment may be necessary for those patients presenting with neurologic and psychiatric manifestations of disease. Patient symptoms and laboratory test levels should be monitored for improvement. If there is no improvement or only minimal improvement, providers should seek alternative disease theories for an explanation of the anemia.

In folic acid deficiency, patients may reveal a history of excessive alcohol intake, poor diet, pregnancy, or chronic use of certain medication, such as methotrexate or sulfonamides. Patients may complain of tongue soreness, dysphagia, or more generalized symptoms of nausea, vomiting, abdominal pain, and fatigue. Physical examination may reveal glossy, beefy appearance of the tongue, angular stomatitis, and hyperpigmentation of mucosal areas as well as palms and soles. Additionally,

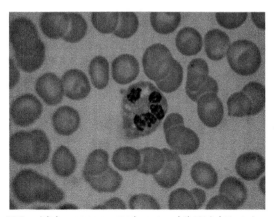

Fig. 6. Macrocytic RBCs with hypersegmented neutrophil. Wright's stain, original magnification 1000×. (*Courtesy of* James A. Van Rhee, MS, PA-C and Jane McDaniel, MS, MLS, SC.)

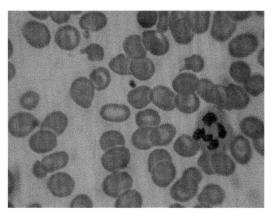

Fig. 7. Hypersegmented neutrophil. Wright's stain, original magnification 1000×. (*Courtesy of* James A. Van Rhee, MS, PA-C and Jane McDaniel, MS, MLS, SC.)

neurologic signs and symptoms, such as various forms of cognitive impairment and other physical manifestations of psychiatric illness, such as depression, may be the initial presenting complaint.

Work-up of folic acid deficiency should be prompted by history and physical examination and should include a CBC, red cell indices, serum vitamin B_{12} level, and serum folate levels as well as serum MMA levels to differentiate the 2 megaloblastic anemias. Treatment of folic acid deficiency should include a varied diet, including leafy greens, fruits, vegetables, and foods fortified with folic acid. Additionally, depending on the level of deficiency, discontinuation of medications causing the deficiency (if any) should be considered; the risks and benefits of discontinuing medications should be conducted on a case-by-case basis. Folic acid, 0.4 mg to 1 mg, should be administered orally, intravenously, intramuscularly, or subcutaneously.[15] The route of administration depends on the setting and presentation of the patient.

SUMMARY

Interpretation of the CBC is a skill that every provider must have facility with. A CBC provides insight into various disease processes and pathologies and, based on patient history, can be a valuable tool in diagnosing anemia. Anemias affect the population on a global scale and, although their presentations may vary, accurate diagnosis and treatment are crucial to improving patient outcomes. A nuanced understanding of the CBC as well the pathophysiology of iron metabolism can help the health care provider educate the patient.

REVIEW
Open-ended Questions

Case A
A 28-year-old Italian woman presents for a physical examination. She notes occasional mild fatigue and shortness of breath. She is contemplating pregnancy in the upcoming year. She is on no medications and admits to social alcohol use. Her menses are regular, lasting 6 days. She denies gastrointestinal issues. Physical examination reveals mildly pale conjunctiva and negative stool hemoccult. Otherwise, examination is negative.

1. What other questions should be asked on history?
2. Which systems on physical examination should be closely assessed for signs of disease?

3. What types of anemias are on the differential diagnosis list?
4. What laboratory studies should be ordered at this visit?

In this patient, the following laboratory test results return: white blood cell count and platelets are within normal range; however, hemoglobin is low, at 10.7 g/d/L, and hematocrit is 33%. MCV is noted to be 65 fL and MCH is 28 pg. Iron studies reveal a normal serum ferritin, normal serum iron, and normal TIBC.

1. What diagnosis is most likely?
2. Is further testing required for a confirmatory diagnosis?
3. What is the treatment and management of this patient?
4. What education should be provided with regard to her future pregnancy?

Case B
A 75-year-old man presents to the clinic with a complaint of tingling in his fingers for the past 6 months. He notes that he fell approximately 4 months ago, which caused a head injury and forehead laceration. He states he eats regularly but not as much he did when his wife was cooking for him. She passed away 18 months ago. He also admits to drinking several drinks per night to "help him sleep."

1. What further information should be elicited on history?
2. Which systems on physical examination should be closely assessed for signs of disease?
3. What laboratory tests should be ordered for initial work-up?
4. What tests should be ordered to confirm the suspected diagnosis?
5. What education should be provided to the patient with regard to his diagnosis?

REFERENCES

1. Fauci A, Braunwald E, Kasper D, et al. Harrisons principles of internal medicine: self-assessment and board review, vol. 59. New York: McGraw-Hill Education; 2018.
2. South-Paul JE, Matheny SC, Lewis EL, editors. CURRENT diagnosis & treatment: family medicine, vol. 32, 4th edition. New York: McGraw-Hill; 2015. Available at: http://accessmedicine.mhmedical.com/content.aspx?bookid=1415&sectionid=7702250.
3. Hematology complete blood count (CBC). Liver Cirrhosis. Available at: http://www.meddean.luc.edu/lumen/meded/medicine/medclerk/2004_05/level1/cbcanemia/cbclesson.htm. Accessed September 6, 2018.
4. Rossi E. Hepcidin - the iron regulatory hormone. Clin Biochem Rev 2005;26(3):47–9.
5. Porteus M, Mantanona T. Blood. In: Janson LW, Tischler ME. editors. The big picture: medical biochemistry. New York: McGraw-Hill. Available at: http://accessmedicine.mhmedical.com/content.aspx?bookid=2355&sectionid=185845059. Accessed September 06, 2018.
6. Waldvogel-Abramowski S, Waeber G, Gassner C, et al. Physiology of iron metabolism. Transfus Med Hemother 2014;41(3):213–21.
7. Siah CW, Ombiga J, Adams LA, et al. Normal iron metabolism and the pathophysiology of iron overload disorders. Clin Biochem Rev 2006;27(1):5–16.
8. Iron deficiency anemia: practice essentials, background, pathophysiology. background, pathophysiology, etiology. 2018. Available at: https://emedicine.medscape.com/article/202333-overview#a5.
9. Kelly AU, Mcsorley ST, Patel P, et al. Interpreting iron studies. BMJ 2017. https://doi.org/10.1136/bmj.j2513.

10. Transferrin saturation: reference range, interpretation, collection and panels. Background, pathophysiology, etiology. 2017. Available at: https://emedicine. medscape.com/article/2087960-overview#showall. Accessed September 6, 2018.
11. Alpha thalassemia treatment & management: approach considerations, iron and folic acid supplementation, general supportive care. Background, pathophysiology, etiology. 2017. Available at: https://emedicine.medscape.com/article/955496-treatment#showall. Accessed September 6, 2018.
12. Cao A, Galanello R. Beta-thalassemia. Genet Med 2010;12(2):61–76. https://doi.org/10.1097/gim.0b013e3181cd68ed.
13. Kaushansky K, Lichtman MA, Prchal JT, et al, editors. Williams hematology, vol. 37, 9th edition. New York: McGraw-Hill; 2016. Available at: http://accessmedicine.mhmedical.com/content.aspx?bookid=1581&sectionid=9430114. Accessed September 06, 2018.
14. Fraenkel PG. Understanding anemia of chronic disease. Hematology 2015;2015(1):14–8.
15. Megaloblastic anemia: practice essentials, pathophysiology, etiology. Background, pathophysiology, etiology. 2018. Available at: https://emedicine.medscape.com/article/204066-overview#showall. Accessed September 6, 2018.
16. Bunn H, Heeney MM. Iron homeostasis: deficiency and overload. In: Aster JC, Bunn H, editors. Pathophysiology of blood disorders, 2nd edition. New York: McGraw-Hill. Available at: http://accessmedicine.mhmedical.com/content.aspx?bookid=1900&sectionid=137394788. Accessed September 06, 2018.

Hemolytic Anemia
Mass Destruction

James A. Van Rhee, MS, PA-C

KEYWORDS

- Hemolytic anemia • Nonimmune hemolytic anemia • Immune hemolytic anemia

KEY POINTS

- Hemolytic anemias may be acute or chronic and life-threatening. They should be considered in all patients with an unexplained normocytic or macrocytic anemia.
- Hemolytic anemias can be divided into acquired or congenital.
- A detailed history and focused laboratory evaluation are necessary to properly evaluate a patient with a possible hemolytic anemia.

INTRODUCTION

Hemolytic anemia is defined by the premature destruction of red blood cells (RBCs). Hemolytic anemia may be acute or chronic and life-threatening, and it should be considered in all patients with a normocytic or macrocytic anemia that is unexplained. Hemolytic anemias present with laboratory evidence of increased red cell destruction, suggested by elevation in lactate dehydrogenase (LDH); increased hemoglobin breakdown, suggested by increase in indirect bilirubin; decreased level of haptoglobin; and an increase in bone marrow erythropoiesis, suggested by an increase in reticulocytes.

PATHOPHYSIOLOGY

Premature destruction of RBCs can be intravascular or extravascular in the monocyte-macrophage system of the spleen and liver; extravascular destruction is more common. The primary extravascular mechanism is through sequestration of RBCs and phagocytosis due to RBCs' inability to deform. The mechanism of antibody-mediated hemolysis is via phagocytosis or complement-mediated destruction and can occur intravascular or extravascular. The intravascular mechanisms include direct cellular destruction via lysis, toxins, or trauma; fragmentation, when shearing or rupture of the RBCs occurs; and oxidation, when the protective mechanisms of the cells are unable to the protect the RBCs from destruction.[1]

Disclosure Statement: Nothing to disclose.
Yale Physician Assistant Online Program, Yale School of Medicine, 100 Church Street South, Suite A230, New Haven, CT 06519, USA
E-mail address: james.vanrhee@yale.edu

Physician Assist Clin 4 (2019) 649–662
https://doi.org/10.1016/j.cpha.2019.02.012
2405-7991/19/© 2019 Elsevier Inc. All rights reserved.

The etiologies of hemolysis are numerous and mechanisms include the following (**Table 1**):

- Hemoglobinopathies, such as sickle cell disease, which lead to splenic destruction via multiple mechanisms
- Membrane disorders, such as hereditary spherocytosis (HS), due to inherited protein deficits leading to increased destruction
- Enzyme deficiencies, such as glucose-6-phosphate dehydrogenase (G6PD) deficiency, secondary to hemolysis due to oxidative stress or decreased energy production in the cell
- Immune-mediated hemolytic anemia, in which antibodies bind with the RBCs resulting in phagocytosis or complement-mediated destruction
- Extrinsic nonimmune causes, such as microangiopathic hemolytic anemia (MAHA), infections, direct trauma, and drug-induced hemolysis, resulting in fragmentation of the RBCs

CLINICAL PRESENTATION

The clinical presentation of hemolytic anemias is variable and nonspecific. Acute hemolytic anemia should be considered in a patient who presents with acute jaundice or

Table 1
Etiologies of hemolytic anemia

Etiology	Example	Mechanism	Vascular Location
AIHA	Warm or cold autoantibodies	Splenic trapping, phagocytosis, complement activation	Extravascular or intravascular
Drug induced	Drug-induced TMA, drug-induced immune hemolytic anemia	Direct, toxin, phagocytosis, fragmentation	Extravascular or intravascular
Enzymopathy	G6PD or PK deficiencies	Oxidative lysis	Intravascular
Hemoglobinopathy	Sickle cell disease, hemoglobin C disease	Splenic trapping	Extravascular
Infection	Malaria, *Babesia*, Clostridia	Direct, toxin, phagocytosis, fragmentation	Extravascular or intravascular
Membrane structural abnormalities	HS, HE, paroxysmal nocturnal hemoglobinuria	Splenic trapping	Extravascular
MAHA	TTP, HUS, disseminated intravascular coagulation, HELLP syndrome, drug-induced TMA	Fragmentation	Intravascular
Systemic disease	Hypertensive emergencies, systemic lupus erythematosus, scleroderma, liver disease, hypersplenism	Splenic trapping, fragmentation	Extravascular or intravascular
Trauma	Endovascular devices, aortic stenosis, extracorporeal membrane oxygenation, arteriovenous malformation, burns	Fragmentation, direct trauma	Intravascular

hematuria in the presence of anemia. The clinical presentation of patients with chronic hemolytic anemia includes lymphadenopathy, hepatosplenomegaly, cholestasis, and choledocholithiasis. Other nonspecific symptoms include fatigue, dyspnea, hypotension, chest pain, and tachycardia.

EVALUATION

Fig. 1 provides an overview of the work-up of patients with a hemolytic anemia. The first step in the evaluation of a patient with hemolytic anemia is to determine if the hemolytic anemia is acquired or congenital. Does the patient have a personal or family history of anemia? If so, a congenital etiology is possible. When hemolysis is suspected, a complete history should be obtained, including past medical history, medications, social history, family history, and review of systems. The physical examination should focus on identifying underlying etiologies and associated conditions, such as infections, autoimmune disease, and malignancies (**Table 2**).

The initial laboratory work-up of the patient with hemolytic anemia should begin with a complete blood cell count. Evaluate for anemia and then classify the anemia as normocytic (mean corpuscular volume between 80 fL and 100 fL) or macrocytic (mean corpuscular volume >100 fL). Once an anemia is identified other tests that should be obtained include evaluation of the peripheral blood smear, reticulocyte count, LDH level, haptoglobin, unconjugated bilirubin levels, and a urinalysis (**Table 3**).

- LDH is intracellular and increased levels are noted in hemolysis of RBCs.
- Haptoglobin is a protein that binds to free hemoglobin in the circulation, and levels are decreased in RBC hemolysis.

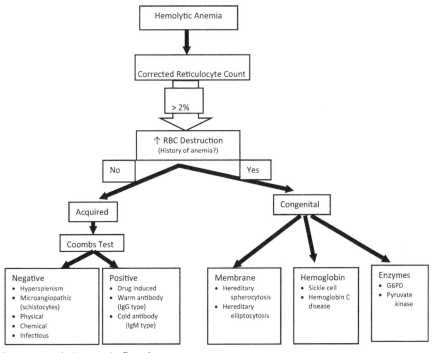

Fig. 1. Hemolytic anemia flowchart.

Table 2
History and physical examination findings

History and Physical Examination Findings	Possible Etiologies
Acute-onset jaundice	All hemolytic anemias
Diarrhea	HUS (*Escherichia coli* O157:H7)
Fever, chills	AIHA, disseminated intravascular coagulation, HUS, infection (malaria, *Babesia*)
Hematuria	Paroxysmal nocturnal hemoglobinuria, intravascular hemolysis
History of malignancy	Warm autoantibody hemolytic anemia
Medications	Drug-induced TMA anemia, drug-induced immune hemolytic anemia, G6PD deficiency
Positive family history of hemolytic anemia	Sickle cell disease, HS, HE, G6PD deficiency, PK deficiency
Recent infection with Epstein-Barr virus or *Mycoplasma pneumoniae*	Cold autoantibody hemolytic anemia

- Unconjugated bilirubin levels rise as its production exceeds elimination capability.
- Increase in reticulocytes is noted in RBC hemolysis leading to macrocytic RBCs, unless another etiology for the anemia, such as iron deficiency or bone marrow suppression is present. The reticulocyte should be corrected for the degree of anemia to ensure that the degree of reticulocytosis is adequate.
- Urinalysis may be positive for hemoglobinuria in hemolytic anemia despite no visible RBCs on microscopic examination of the urine.

The presence of increased reticulocytes, elevated LDH, elevated unconjugated bilirubin, and decreased haptoglobin levels confirms the presence of hemolysis. The absence of these findings should lead to the evaluation of other possible causes of the anemia.

Examining the peripheral blood smear is important in identifying the specific etiology of various hemolytic anemias. The peripheral blood should be examined for the presence of spherocytes, schistocytes, sickle cells, bite cells, or blister cells.

- Spherocytes are caused by membrane deficits or repeated small membrane removals by macrophages (**Fig. 2**).

Table 3
Initial laboratory tests for hemolysis

Test	Finding in Hemolysis	Cause
Haptoglobin	Decreased	Binds free hemoglobin
LDH	Elevated	Released from lysis of RBCs
Peripheral blood smear	Abnormal RBCs	Based on cause of anemia
Reticulocyte count	Increased	Marrow response to anemia
Unconjugated bilirubin	Increased	Increased hemoglobin breakdown
Urinalysis	Presence of urobilinogen and blood	Free hemoglobin and its metabolites

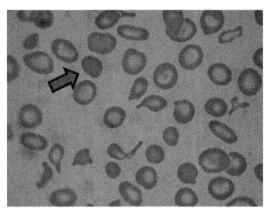

Fig. 2. Spherocytes noted in hemolytic anemia. Wright's stain, original magnification 1000x. (*Courtesy of* James A. Van Rhee MS, PA-C and Jane McDaniel, MS, MLS, SC.)

- Schistocytes are fragmented cells that result from intravascular destruction (**Fig. 3**).
- Sickle cells are elongated cells and occur when hypoxia leads to the development of rigid protein strands in the RBCs, causing a change in cell shape (**Fig. 4**).
- Bite and blister cells result from partial phagocytosis and occur in oxidative causes of anemia (**Fig. 5**).

The direct antiglobulin test (DAT), or direct Coombs test, further differentiates immune hemolytic anemia from nonimmune causes. In a patient with an acquired hemolytic anemia, the DAT is used to determine whether the RBCs have surface bound immunoglobulin G (IgG) and/or complement. The main use of the DAT is to determine if the hemolysis is immune dependent or immune independent. The underlying mechanism of the DAT is that antihuman globulin (AHG) agglutinates antibody-coated cells. Testing starts with polyspecific AHG containing both anti-IgG and anticomplement and then any positive results are repeated with monospecific AHG to individually detect IgG or complement[2] (**Fig. 6**).

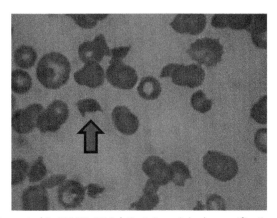

Fig. 3. Schistocytes noted in MAHA. Wright's stain, original magnification 1000x. (*Courtesy of* James A. Van Rhee MS, PA-C and Jane McDaniel, MS, MLS, SC.)

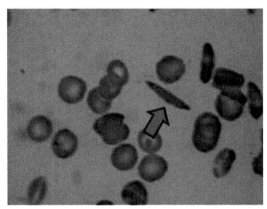

Fig. 4. Sickle cell noted in sickle cell anemia. Wright's stain, original magnification 1000x. (*Courtesy of* James A. Van Rhee MS, PA-C and Jane McDaniel, MS, MLS, SC.)

IMMUNE HEMOLYTIC ANEMIA
Autoimmune Hemolytic Anemia

Autoimmune hemolytic anemia (AIHA) is caused by autoantibody-mediated destruction. The classic laboratory finding is a positive DAT. AIHA is organized into 2 subgroups based on the binding temperatures of the autoantibody, either cold or warm agglutinins. Many cases of AIHA are idiopathic; however, viral and bacterial infections, autoimmune conditions, connective tissue disorder, lymphoproliferative malignancies, and blood transfusions are associated with AIHA.

Warm autoantibodies are more common than cold autoantibodies and involve IgG antibodies that react with the RBC membrane at normal body temperatures. These RBCs, coated with IgG, are then removed by reticuloendothelial macrophages in the spleen and sequestered in the spleen, which can lead to splenomegaly. First-line treatment of warm autoantibodies is glucocorticoids, with a response noted in 70% to 85% of patients and curative in 20% to 30% of cases.[3] Second lines of therapy include splenectomy, rituximab, and other immunosuppressive drugs, such as azathioprine and cyclophosphamide. Management also should include treatment of the underlying condition, blood transfusions as needed, and supportive care.

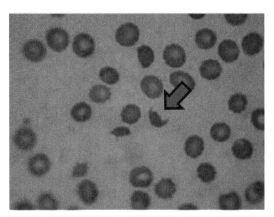

Fig. 5. Bite cells noted in G6PD deficiency. Wright's stain, original magnification 1000x. (*Courtesy of* James A. Van Rhee MS, PA-C and Jane McDaniel, MS, MLS, SC.)

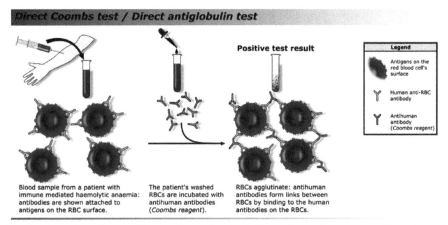

Fig. 6. Direct Coombs test. (*From* Wikimedia. Available at: https://commons.wikimedia.org/w/index.php?curid=517391.)

Cold autoantibodies involve IgM antibodies. These autoantibodies react at low temperatures, with antigens on the RBC surface leading to RBC cell lysis on rewarming via complement fixation causing intravascular hemolysis. Primary chronic cold agglutinin disease accounts for 15% of all cases and should be suspected in elderly patients with chronic hemolytic anemia, symptoms such as Raynaud phenomenon, and agglutination of RBCs on peripheral blood smear. Development of these cold autoantibodies also is associated with secondary cold agglutinin disease due to infections, such as mycoplasma pneumonia and infectious mononucleosis, or malignant processes. Treatment consists of supportive measures, avoidance of triggers, and management of the underlying disease. Recent studies have shown that the combination of fludarabine and rituximab or rituximab alone can be effective in treating patients with cold agglutinin disease.[4] Corticosteroids should not be used to treat primary cold agglutinin disease.

Drug-induced Immune Hemolytic Anemia

Drug-induced immune hemolytic anemia is a rare occurrence that results from drug-induced antibodies. The most common drug groups causing an immune hemolytic anemia include antimicrobials (42%), nonsteroidal anti-inflammatory drugs (16%), anti-neoplastic medications (13%), and antihypertensives (6%).[5] There are 3 common mechanisms of drug-induced immune hemolytic anemia (**Table 4**).

Table 4
Drug-induced immune hemolytic anemia

Mechanism	Hapten	Immune Complex	Autoantibody
DAT	Positive	Positive	Positive
Anti-IgG	Positive	Rarely positive	Positive
Anti-C3d	Rarely positive	Positive	Negative
Indirect Coombs (drug not in system)	Negative	Negative	Either
Indirect Coombs (drug in system)	Positive	Positive	No change
Examples	Cephalothin Ampicillin Methicillin	*Hydrochlorothiazide* Antihistamines Rifampin/isoniazid Sulfonamides Quinidine	Levodopa Ibuprofen Diclofenac α-Interferon Methyldopa

- Hapten induced—in which the drug, which is the hapten, binds to the RBC membrane and antibodies are now made directed against the hapten.
- Immune complex—antibody is produced against part-drug, part-RBC membrane components.
- Autoantibody—antibody is produced against membrane components, producing a reaction similar to that of autoimmune disease.

The DAT is positive in patients with drug-induced immune hemolytic anemia. Currently, cefotetan, ceftriaxone, piperacillin (in combination piperacillin/tazobactam), and nonsteroidal anti-inflammatory drugs predominate. The progression of this condition typically is gradual, and treatment involves removal of the offending agent and RBC transfusion as needed.

NONIMMUNE HEMOLYTIC ANEMIA–ACQUIRED
Microangiopathic Hemolytic Anemia

MAHA is hemolytic anemia that occurs when RBCs fragment and results in schistocytes on the peripheral blood smear. This can be caused by trauma from an endovascular device or microthrombi. Thrombotic microangiopathies (TMAs) are a group of clinical entities that share MAHA as a key feature. Two of the major TMAs are thrombotic thrombocytopenic purpura (TTP) and hemolytic uremic syndrome.

Thrombotic Thrombocytopenic Purpura

TTP is characterized by thrombocytopenia, fever, renal injury, presence of schistocytes, and neurologic dysfunction. This presentation has significant overlap with the presentation of hemolytic uremic syndrome (HUS); however, HUS typically has more renal injury and less neurologic dysfunction. Now TTP can be better diagnosed by noting a significantly reduced ADAMTS13 enzyme activity. The ADAMTS13 enzyme cleaves von Willebrand factor aggregations and, when this ADAMTS13 enzyme is lacking or nonfunctional, large von Willebrand factor multimers form. These multimers trap platelets, leading to the development of microthrombi and RBC destruction by shearing the RBCs, creating schistocytes.

TTP is life threatening and requires timely diagnosis and treatment. Additional laboratory findings include a negative DAT result and normal coagulation testing. Assessment of ADAMTS13 enzyme activity is diagnostic for TTP, but making a presumptive diagnosis based on clinical presentation and basic laboratory tests is important. Once a presumptive diagnosis is made, immediate treatment with plasma exchange and glucocorticoids should be started. Plasma exchange removes affected platelets and autoantibodies while replenishing ADAMTS13 enzyme levels.

Hemolytic Uremic Syndrome

HUS is characterized by MAHA, acute kidney injury, thrombocytopenia, and neurologic dysfunction. HUS can be separated from TTP based on ADAMTS13 enzyme activity. HUS is caused most commonly by a Shiga toxin producing *Escherichia coli* (STEC) HUS, accounting for 90% of cases, and is also caused by STEC organisms, such as O157:H7 and *Shigella dysenteriae*.[6] The primary source of STEC infection is inadequately cooked ground beef, but fruits, vegetables, poultry, and contaminated drinking water also have been implicated. It most commonly affects children and presents with abdominal pain with diarrhea, following 5 days to 10 days later with MAHA, acute kidney injury, and thrombocytopenia. *Streptococcus pneumoniae,* HIV, and influenza also have been associated with HUS in rare cases and present without the classic prodrome. Treatment of STEC-HUS is supportive care and continued evaluation of renal function. Antibiotics are not recommended for gastrointestinal STEC because they may increase the risk of HUS.[7] Eculizumab has been shown effective in the treatment of HUS.[8]

Other Microangiopathic Hemolytic Anemia Syndromes

Other clinical entities that cause MAHA include hemolysis, elevated liver enzymes, and low platelet count (HELLP) syndrome and disseminated intravascular coagulation. HELLP syndrome is related to pregnancy and shares many of the same characteristics of TTP and HUS. TTP and HUS do not usually induce liver enzyme elevations as in HELLP syndrome.[9] A low LDH–to–aspartate transaminase ratio can aid in distinguishing HELLP syndrome, because the rate of hemolysis is higher in the other TMAs and hepatic involvement is higher in HELLP syndrome.[10] Disseminated intravascular coagulation also can result in MAHA due to fibrin-rich microthrombi. Disseminated intravascular coagulation causes thrombocytopenia, prolonged coagulation studies, positive D-dimer test results, decreased fibrinogen levels, and elevated fibrinogen degradation products.[11]

Drug-induced Thrombotic Microangiopathy

Drug-induced TMA occurs when a medication causes the formation of platelet microthrombi, resulting in MAHA through induced antibodies or direct toxicity. These antibodies interact only in the presence of the drug. The clinical features are similar to those of other MAHA syndromes. In a 2015 review, the overall incidence of drug-induced TMA was 5% of all MAHA cases.[12] Quinine, cyclosporine, and tacrolimus made up more than 50% of all drug-induced TMA cases.[13] The management of drug-induced TMA includes discontinuing the offending agent and providing supportive care; plasma exchange is not beneficial, except in the cases involving ticlopidine.

Other etiologies include hypersplenism, physical, and infectious etiologies. Hypersplenism is the increased pooling and or destruction of RBCs by the enlarged spleen. Splenomegaly is noted in hypersplenism and is characterized by a reduction in 1 or more of the blood's cellular elements in the presence of normocellular or hypercellular bone marrow. Most cases of anemia secondary to hypersplenism are asymptomatic. Physical etiologies include burns, snake venom, and toxic chemicals.

Infectious etiologies include malaria, *Babesia*, and *Clostridium perfringens*. Malaria, caused by various species of *Plasmodium*, is the most common etiology of hemolytic anemia in the world. Symptoms include fever, splenomegaly, hemolytic anemia, and thrombocytopenia. The anemia typically is normocytic and normochromic, and increased reticulocytes may not be noted secondary to suppression of erythropoietic precursors. Diagnosis is made by observation of the parasite in the RBCs on blood films. *Babesia* are an intraerythrocytic protozoa transmitted by ticks. Diagnosis is made by examination of blood smear and serology.

NONIMMUNE HEMOLYTIC ANEMIA–CONGENITAL

The congenital hemolytic anemias typically present in infancy or early childhood. The family history may be positive for hemolytic anemia, and infants may have significant hyperbilirubinemia. Patients present with pallor, jaundice, and possibly splenomegaly. Laboratory studies reveal a reticulocytosis, elevated indirect bilirubin, and abnormalities on peripheral blood smear and are DAT negative (**Table 5**).

Membrane Disorders

HS is due to protein mutations involved in the interactions between the lipid bilayer and spectrin-based cytoskeleton on the RBC membrane. This mutation leads to a

Table 5
Peripheral blood smear findings congenital hemolytic anemia

Disease	Polychromasia	Spherocytes	Elliptocytes	Heinz Bodies	Sickle Cells
HS	X	X	—	—	—
Hereditary elliptocytosis	X	—	X	—	—
G6PG deficiency	X	—	—	X	—
PK deficiency	X	—	—	—	—
Sickle cell anemia	X	—	—	—	X

loss of RBC surface area and the formation of a spherocyte (see **Fig. 2**). HS is an autosomal dominant disorder and is most commonly noted in people of northern European ancestry; 1 in 2000 people in northern Europe and North America are affected.[14] Patients present with pallor, splenomegaly, and jaundice; laboratory testing reveals spherocytes on peripheral blood smear, increased reticulocytes, and a negative DAT. The osmotic fragility test is considered the gold standard for diagnosing HS but is falsely negative in approximately 25% of patients.[15] Recent guidelines recommend eosin-5-maleimide (EMA) binding test as the appropriate screening test.[16] EMA binding is deficient in HS. Treatment includes splenectomy, which reduces hemolysis; splenectomy is indicated in moderate to severe disease. Cholecystectomy should be considered at the time of splenectomy as gallstone development is common in patients with chronic hemolysis.

Hereditary elliptocytosis (HE) is the second most common membrane disorder, behind HS. In HE, the RBCs are elliptical or oval in shape (**Fig. 7**) and result from defects in the protein connection in the RBC membrane. HE is autosomal dominant and affects 3 to 5 people per 10,000 population.[17] Most patients are asymptomatic, but neonates can present with jaundice, hemolysis, and hydrops fetalis.[17] Patients with severe disease should be considered for splenectomy.

Hemoglobin Disorders

Sickle cell anemia is an inherited disorder caused by a point mutation leading to a substitution of valine for glutamic acid in position 6 of the beta chain of hemoglobin. Membrane abnormalities from sickling and oxidative damage caused by hemoglobin S,

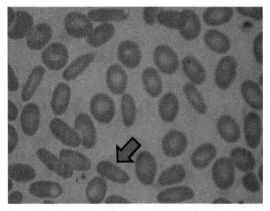

Fig. 7. Elliptocytes found in heredity elliptocytosis. Wright's stain, original magnification 1000x. (*Courtesy of* James A. Van Rhee MS, PA-C and Jane McDaniel, MS, MLS, SC.)

along with impaired deformability of sickle cells, leads to splenic trapping and removal of cells. Some degree of intravascular hemolysis occurs as well. Sickle cell disease is more common in certain ethnic groups, including people of African descent, including African Americans, Hispanic Americans from Central and South America, and people of Middle Eastern, Asian, Indian, and Mediterranean descent. Sickle cell disease symptoms typically appear by 4 months of age. Symptoms include pallor, jaundice, bone pain, edema, and recurrent painful episodes and chronic organ disease secondary to vaso-occlusion. Laboratory testing reveals sickle cells on peripheral blood smear and hemoglobin electrophoresis reveals a predominance of hemoglobin S. Treatment consists of immunizations for *S pneumoniae*, *Haemophilus influenzae*, hepatitis B, and influenza.

Hemoglobin C disease is one-fourth as frequent as sickle cell disease among African Americans. Laboratory testing reveals mild anemia and mild reticulocytosis. The predominant RBC abnormality on the peripheral smear is an abundance of target cells, and crystal-containing cells also may be seen (**Fig. 8**). Splenomegaly may be the only physical finding, and the frequency of acute painful episodes is approximately half that found in sickle cell disease, with a life expectancy 2 decades longer.[18] Significant morbidity, however, can occur. The incidence of fatal bacterial infection is less than in sickle cell anemia, but there is an increased risk of *S pneumoniae* and *H influenzae* infection.

Enzyme Disorders

Oxidative hemolysis occurs when normal processes are unable to reduce ferric iron, also known as methemoglobin, to ferrous iron, which carries oxygen. This results in the denaturing of ferric hemoglobin into multimers, called Heinz bodies, and leads to premature RBC destruction by phagocytosis. G6PD is integral to these protective systems, and, when it is deficient, oxidative insults may cause hemolysis. G6PD deficiency is an X-linked disorder and is common in individuals of Mediterranean and African descent. Classically, fava beans, sulfa drugs, and primaquine were the primary triggers of oxidative hemolysis, but the number of medications to avoid in persons with G6PD deficiency is extensive and listed in **Table 6**. Diagnosis is made by G6PD

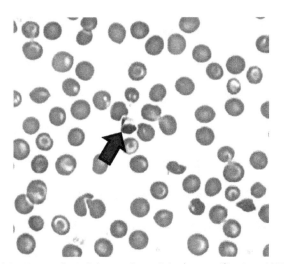

Fig. 8. Hemoglobin C crystal. Wright's stain, original magnification 1000x. (*Courtesy of* James A. Van Rhee MS, PA-C and Jane McDaniel, MS, MLS, SC.)

Table 6
Drug to avoid in glucose-6-phosphate dehydrogenase deficiency

Class	Drug
Analgesics	Acetylsalicylic acid Acetaminophen
Antibiotics	Nitrofurans Quinolones Chloramphenicol Sulfonamides
Anthelmintics	β-Naphthol Niridazole Stibophen
Antimalarials	Mepacrine Pamaquine Pentaquine Primaquine
Antimycobacterial	Dapsone Para-aminosalicylic acid Sulfones
Antineoplastic	Doxorubicin Rasburicase
Cardiovascular drugs	Dopamine Procainamide Quinidine Hydralazine Methyldopa
Genitourinary analgesics	Phenazopyridine
Gout preparations	Colchicine Probenecid
Other	Fava beans Naphthalene

activity testing. Treatment is discontinuation of the drug and supportive care. Methylene blue is indicated for the treatment of severe methemoglobinemia from a non-G6PD cause, but it is possibly harmful and contraindicated in persons with G6PD deficiency.[19]

Pyruvate kinase (PK) deficiency is the most common enzyme deficiency causing hemolysis. The enzyme PK is important in energy generation in the cell. Although it is the second most common enzyme disorder to G6PD deficiency, the vast majority of patients with G6PD deficiency never suffer a hemolytic episode. PK deficiency is noted worldwide but is more common among people of northern European extraction.[20] PK deficiency is an autosomal recessive disease. Splenomegaly often is present, and patients with severe hemolysis may be chronically jaundiced and may develop gallstones, transient aplastic anemia crises, and folate deficiency. Because the hemolysis is extravascular with a variable intravascular hemolysis, increased LDH, hyperbilirubinemia, and low haptoglobin levels may be present. The reticulocyte count increases after splenectomy. RBC morphology is nonspecific in PK deficiency. A screening test using crude hemolysate with a single concentration substrate has been used for the detection of pyruvate deficiency but occasionally misses some PK variants. Specialized laboratories can perform quantitative PK enzyme analysis and further analyze the mutant enzyme by comprehensive kinetic studies.[21] Many patients do not require therapy. Some require RBC transfusions and splenectomy has documented benefit in severe cases.

SUMMARY

Hemolytic anemias may be acute or chronic and life threatening. They should be considered in all patients with an unexplained normocytic or macrocytic anemia. A detailed history should be obtained and basic laboratory test, such as LDH, indirect bilirubin, haptoglobin, and reticulocyte count, and review of the peripheral blood smear should direct the clinician to more specific tests that can aid in the diagnosis.

REFERENCES

1. Mentzer WC, Schrier SL. Extrinsic nonimmune hemolytic anemias. In: Hoffman R, Benz EJ Jr, Silberstein LE, et al, editors. Hematology: basic principles and practice. 7th edition. Philadelphia: Elsevier; 2018. p. 663–72.
2. Zantek ND, Koepsell SA, Tharp DR, et al. The direct antiglobulin test: a critical step in the evaluation of hemolysis. Am J Hematol 2012;87:707–9.
3. Zanella A, Barcellini W. Treatment of autoimmune hemolytic anemias. Haematologica 2014;99:1547–54.
4. Berentsen S. Cold agglutinin disease. Hematology 2016;1:226–31.
5. Garratty G. Immune hemolytic anemia associated with drug therapy. Blood Rev 2010;24:143–50.
6. Ardissino G, Salardi S, Colombo E, et al. Epidemiology of haemolytic uremic syndrome in children. Data from the North Italian HUS network. Eur J Pediatr 2016; 175:465–73.
7. Wong CS, Jelacic S, Habeeb RL, et al. The risk of the hemolytic-uremic syndrome after antibiotic treatment of Escherichia coli O157:H7 infections. N Engl J Med 2000;342:1930–6.
8. Legendre CM, Licht C, Muus P, et al. Terminal complement inhibitor eculizumab in atypical hemolytic-uremic syndrome. N Engl J Med 2013;368:2169–81.
9. Pourrat O, Coudroy R, Pierre F. Differentiation between severe HELLP syndrome and thrombotic microangiopathy, thrombotic thrombocytopenic purpura and other imitators. Eur J Obstet Gynecol Reprod Biol 2015;189:68–72.
10. Keiser SD, Boyd KW, Rehberg JF, et al. A high LDH to AST ratio helps to differentiate pregnancy-associated thrombotic thrombocytopenic purpura (TTP) from HELLP syndrome. J Matern Fetal Neonatal Med 2012;25:1059–63.
11. Wada H, Matsumoto T, Yamashita Y. Diagnosis and treatment of disseminated intravascular coagulation (DIC) according to four DIC guidelines. J Intensive Care 2014;2:15.
12. Reese JA, Bougie DW, Curtis BR, et al. Drug-induced thrombotic microangiopathy: experience of the Oklahoma Registry and the Blood Center of Wisconsin. Am J Hematol 2015;90:406–10.
13. Al-Nouri ZL, Reese JA, Terrell DR, et al. Drug-induced thrombotic microangiopathy: a systematic review of published reports. Blood 2015;125:616–8.
14. Perrotta S, Gallagher PG, Mohandas N. Hereditary spherocytosis. Lancet 2008; 372:1411–26.
15. Bianchi P, Fermo E, Vercellati C, et al. Diagnostic power of laboratory tests for hereditary spherocytosis: a comparison study of 150 patients grouped according to molecular abd clinical characteristics. Haematologica 2012;97(4):516–23.
16. Bolton-Maggs PH, Langer JC, Iolascon A, et al. General haematology task force of the British committee for standards in haematology: guidelines for the

diagnosis and management of hereditary spherocytosis-2011 update. Br J Haematol 2012;156(1):37–49.

17. Gallagher PG, Weed SA, Tse WT, et al. Recurrent fatal hydrops fetalis associated with a nucleotide substitution in the erythrocyte beta-spectrin gene. J Clin Invest 1995;95(3):1174–82.

18. Platt OS, Brambilla DJ, Rosse WF, et al. Mortality in sickle cell disease. Life expectancy and risk factors for early death. N Engl J Med 1994;330:1639.

19. Sikka P, Bindra VK, Kapoor S, et al. Blue cures blue but be cautious. J Pharm Bio-Allied Sci 2011;3:543–5.

20. Zanella A, Bianchi P. Red cell pyruvate kinase deficiency: from genetics to clinical manifestations. Best Pract Res Clin Haematol 2000;13(1):57–81.

21. Prchal JY, Gregg XT. Red cell enzymes. Hematology Am Soc Hematol Educ Program 2005;1:19–23.

Printed and bound by CPI Group (UK) Ltd, Croydon, CR0 4YY

03/10/2024

01040399-0018